T0192411

THE VALUES
OF PSYCHOTHERAPY

THE VALUES
OF PSYCHOTHERAPY

Jeremy Holmes   *Richard Lindley*

Revised Edition

Foreword by
R. D. Hinshelwood

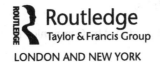

Routledge
Taylor & Francis Group

LONDON AND NEW YORK

Originally published 1989 by Oxford University Press

Fist published in 1998 by Karnac Books Ltd.

Published 2018 by Routledge
2 Park Square, Milton Park, Abingdon, Oxon OX14 4RN
711 Third Avenue, New York, NY 10017, USA

Routledge is an imprint of the Taylor & Francis Group, an informa business

British Library Cataloguing in Publication Data

A C.I.P. records for this book is available from the British Library.

ISBN 9781855751514 (pbk)

Edited, designed, and produced by Comminication Crafts

For El and Ros

CONTENTS

FOREWORD

R. D. Hinshelwood

There is no objectivity in the human sciences. Psychotherapy is one research field that has really addressed that fact. It is accepted that the psychotherapist profoundly affects the field of study whilst in the process of studying it—and the researcher goes on creating an unfolding effect as long as it lasts. The therapeutic effect is, of course, founded on just the same view too: the field of study (the patient or client) is deeply affected by the researcher in a persistent, on-going manner.

But, more than this, there is another and comparable mutual influence: psychotherapy and society also influence each other in a two-way fashion. The Western world has not been left untouched by the coming of Freud (and, to a lesser extent, Janet and nineteenth-century hypnotherapies). Psychotherapy has led to a widely accepted change in our understanding of what a person is. Our sense of our-selves and of how we relate to each other is, in part, a product of the century of psychotherapy, just as psychotherapy is, in part, the creation of the historical development of our society. The values of psychotherapy are, in a deep sense, the values of society in general.

I was very grateful during my own researches when the first edition of this book appeared in 1989. Though my own ideas eventually developed in a somewhat divergent way, it was in no small measure because of the stimulus that this book gives to our thinking about the nature and place of personal autonomy. No single ethical concept has complete hegemony, but in our present times, increasingly, that of autonomy is "more equal than the others". Of course, what psychotherapy means by autonomy is not quite the same as our consumerist society's idea of it. The latter, consumerism, means the freedom to choose what material things to buy and possess. The psychotherapist, on the other hand, looks inward—a quite different direction. His work is to enable the individual person to take possession of his inward things—to own his anger, his jealousy, and so on. These, too, are his possessions. But, whichever—inwards or outwards—the person and his possessions, and his freedom amongst them, are the values of our times.

Consequently, to this extent, psychotherapy is two-faced. It drives a conformist thrust towards the notion of a freedom for the individual. This makes psychotherapy congenial to Western society, provided that the actual nature of the freedom is not looked at too closely. On the other hand, psychotherapy is subversive. It attempts implicitly to recognize that there are (or may be) riches greater than material ones—the inward riches of personal integration, of sincerity of relationships. It is pinpointing this exactly—making explicit this implicit recognition—that makes this a great book.

This volume does not make a plea for the values of psychotherapy—or, at least, that is not where its main importance lies. Instead, it subjects these values to a clarity of vision that, in turn, allows a clearer social debate about them, and about the place of psychotherapy in society. That achievement, of displaying the implicit, is the psychotherapist's true aim. We might call it the task of enhancing autonomy, but equally it is the task of displaying a fuller knowledge of the alternatives that we have as individuals and as a society. It is the task of knowledge itself.

Knowledge is the value of psychotherapy. But this concept is radical, since we also assume that psychotherapy is about happiness, and yet knowledge is not about happiness. Psychotherapy is about knowing oneself, and, unfortunately, that is invariably about disappointment. It is, crucially, the knowledge of unhappiness. Happiness is not the value of psychotherapy.

Freud mused sourly about making neurotic misery into ordinary unhappiness. We might all feel a bit sour about this; no one wants to be unhappy, but who wants to be ordinary either! As the jaded

American tycoon said—"I've been rich and unhappy, and I've been poor and unhappy. And rich is better." External riches do make a difference. As this book conveys, knowledge is about power, or at least the power of personal autonomy. These are internal "riches", and the claim is that they, too, make a difference.

Given these complex evaluations of knowledge and happiness, of inner and outer riches, it is no wonder that there is profound ambivalence in social reactions to psychotherapy. We find a fascination and a suspicion: the hope that it gains us entrance to the real soul of humanity, and contempt that it subverts us by indulgence; our belief in its promise of happiness, and its insistence that we discover something more than happiness.

By now, you may be wondering what sort of beast psychotherapy is. Well, this book gives a fine description. Above all, psychotherapy is a moral practice. However scientific its research, or however much scientific research is demanded of it, psychotherapy remains a practice born of moral dilemmas, of how we live together, each with the other.

And it is the most engaging of all moral practices. For it is three-fold—it is not just that professional, ethical conduct is required of us, as in any other profession; nor is it *just* that its aim is precisely to study the way these two people are together. In addition to these, it is an investigation of the patient's own moral system of values. This book shows that the essence of psychotherapy is an ethical study. That a whole book needs to, and can, be written on the values of psychotherapy is testimony to the fact that psychotherapy is both an investigation and the practice of a moral life.

Above all, the book is a plea to accept psychotherapy as a profession—a new profession that has a claim on the respect and the resources of society around us. The authors claim the support of the National Health Service. Yet, something smacks of special pleading here. There is a sense of being in two minds about grabbing at the coat-tails of the established professions of medicine, nursing, psychology. We could equally say that, as a maturational endeavour, psychotherapy has a claim on educational resources—as the old system of child guidance did. In other words, do we really need to think of our own development as human beings in the same mode as we think of the decline of our bodies in physical illness?

What psychotherapy might demand to be, therefore, is a "National Maturity Service", no less! None of us is a perfect master in the right and wrong ways of conducting ourselves with each other. And to be sure, no psychotherapist is a teacher in this respect. What psychotherapy offers are the conditions for personal growth. Why should such opportunities be limited only to those who are designated as stunted in this respect?

Instead, society itself may be in need of a strong injection of new thinking about moral questions. For so long, science has risen above the merely human, trying to establish a value-neutral territory for itself. That mistake is now coming home to roost, with the need for ethical commissions to investigate the new reproductive technologies, the impact of molecular biology, and even the gestural incorporation of directors of ethics into multinational corporations. This is a broad sweep of the contemporary social landscape. But it is surely not too far-fetched to imagine, at least, the coming together of these elements in something that is not a moral authority, but an authority for moral responsibilities.

Or perhaps that is too far-fetched. What we are invited to do by the forward-looking direction of this book is to imagine the future of psychotherapy. To my mind, that is to imagine the future of the human sciences, emancipated, in part, from the yoke of being a scientific cure. Freed in that way, we see the twenty-first century opening to our visions and ambitions—and not merely to reasons and profit.

January 1998

INTRODUCTION TO THE REVISED EDITION

More than ten years have elapsed since we first set out to write this book. In that time much has changed in the world of psychotherapy. It is gratifying to see that many of the developments that we advocated have come to pass: a determined attempt to establish a profession of psychotherapy; serious consideration of the ethical dilemmas in psychotherapy and how they may be resolved; close scrutiny of psychotherapy trainings and the attempt to introduce standards by which they can be evaluated; recognition of the importance of the spectrum of psychotherapies and of the different contributions each can make to the alleviation of psychological suffering; evaluation of the scientific evidence for and against psychotherapy as a method of treatment (Roth & Fonagy, 1996); a study of the role of psychotherapy within the National Health Service and how it may be effectively enhanced (NHSE, 1996).

We claim no particular credit for these developments: we were simply responding to the *zeitgeist*—psychotherapy is an idea that has finally found its time. In considering a second edition of this book, we worried that events might have overtaken us and that what we said in the 1980s would, a decade later, seem hopelessly dated. But alongside this concern, and in addition to our wish for updating, we felt that there were good reasons for keeping the book alive. First, because we believe that the philosophical underpinnings of our practical arguments remain valid, and merit continued scrutiny. What kind of discipline is psychotherapy—a science, an art, or *sui generis*? Can the goals of psychotherapy be related to the values generally held up as worth striving for within a liberal democracy? Does psychotherapy produce a liberation of the spirit, or merely teach people to conform to the norms of capitalism? What exactly is wrong with sexual relationships between patients and therapists? Are codes of ethics mere professional window-dressing, or can they genuinely protect the public from exploitation by unscrupulous practitioners? These and similar questions continue to be vigorously debated; indeed, philosophical interest in psychotherapy has increased significantly over the past decade (Bloch, 1996).

A second justification for this new edition is that the undoubted advance of psychotherapy has also thrown up new controversies and dilemmas—both practical and political—which need discussion. A good example of the former is the question of False Memories, and whether these can be implanted in patients by over-zealous therapists, or whether this claim is merely part of a general denial of the extent to which sexual abuse exists in our society and of its disastrous psychological effects. A quite different debate centres around the rivalries aroused by the United Kingdom Council for Psychotherapy (UKCP; Clarkson & Pokorny, 1994)—whose establishment has been a major advance towards the professionalization of psychotherapy—and an exclusively psychoanalytical organization, the British Confederation of Psychotherapists (BCP), about who can best represent psychotherapy in the public sphere. The establishment of another organization, Psychotherapists for Social Responsibility, raises the question of the role of psychotherapy in helping to shape social policy (Kraemer & Roberts, 1996). We have tried to tackle these and similar contemporary debates in the new edition.

Preparing a new edition of a book is a tricky job. There is always a course to be steered between complete rewriting (which, no doubt partly out of laziness, we wanted to avoid), and spoiling a good argument by too much tampering. In the end, we used three principles to guide our revision. First, we altered anything that was factually incorrect, whether due to original error or changed circumstances. Second, as mentioned, we have inserted some new discussion of issues that have recently come to the fore. Finally, we have relied on what we have come to call the "wince" criterion: anything that made us blush or wince with embarrassment ("did we really write *that*?") on re-reading was extirpated. We hope our readers are spared too many similar grimaces and may also enjoy or even be enlightened by a subject that for us has lost none of its fascination over the past decade, and will undoubtedly continue to arouse controversy well into the next millennium.

Jeremy Holmes
Richard Lindley
January 1998

PREFACE

C ooperation is the essence of psychotherapy, so it is fitting that the collaboration of which this book is the result has been for both of us so exciting and enjoyable. Despite differing intellectual backgrounds, training, and styles, we have aimed to produce a work which is reasonably unified and coherent. Whether we have succeeded will be for the reader to judge. We certainly feel we have written a far more wide-ranging and generally better book on the subject than either of us could have managed alone.

Since a book is also a collaboration between its readers and the authors, we would like to mention two examples of problems with which we wish to enlist if not the readers' help, then their indulgence. The first is the problem of personal pronouns.

English contains no word meaning "he or she", and it has been customary to use the masculine "he" when "he or she" is intended. To avoid this patriarchal hazard we have used the female "she" (and corresponding "her") as an abbreviation for "he or she" (and "his or hers"), partly because the majority of writers still use "he" and we intend, in a small way, to help restore a balance, partly because it is probably true that the majority of both psychotherapists and psychotherapy patients are women. If this causes offence, we can only apologize, and explicitly repudiate any sexist implications (direct or inverted) of our language.

The second difficulty concerns another troublesome linguistic question: what to call those who receive psychotherapeutic help. Traditionally, psychotherapists and doctors have "patients", counsellors and social workers "clients". This provides opportunities for therapeutic snobbery which is at variance with the spirit of this book (see chapters four and eleven). In the end we decided to stay with the term "patient" for the recipients of psychotherapy, despite the drawback of medical connotations and implied passivity in a process which works best, or perhaps only, when its recipients are actively involved in their own treatment. We have not used "client", partly no doubt because one of us has a medical background, but also because, as we argue in chapter two, psychotherapy is an important form of treatment for those with conditions which are undoubtedly best seen as illnesses. Again, if this terminology causes offence, we crave indulgence.

A word of explanation is needed about the case histories with which we have illustrated the text. Although based on real clinical situations all have been fictionalized either in the interests of confidentiality, or clarity, or both. The exception is the Tarasoff case (see chapter eight) where we have relied on published case material. We are grateful to the patients from whose lives the case histories are derived, and especially where it has not been possible to ask permission to publish, albeit in this disguised form.

A third form of collaboration in the production of any book is that between the authors and their families, friends, and colleagues. The demands for consideration, generosity, support, suggestions, and often very hard work that the writing of a book imposes cannot be underestimated. We would like especially to thank John Baker, Errollyn Bruce, Patricia Bartlett, Roger Fellows, Marj Holmes, Rosamund Holmes, Alison Housley, Peter Lindley, John Lugg, Jonathan Pedder, Oliver Reynolds, Peter Singer, and Lorraine and Robert Tollemache for the help they have given us over the past two years.

Jeremy Holmes
Richard Lindley
December 1988

THE VALUES
OF PSYCHOTHERAPY

CHAPTER ONE

Taking psychotherapy seriously

THE ANXIOUS WIDOW

A farmer's wife in her 30s consulted her doctor, complaining of feelings of panic and doom. She was referred to a psychiatrist. He, a humane and well-trained professional, asked her several questions about her state of mind, satisfied himself that she was not hearing voices or deluded, and sent her back to her doctor with a diagnosis of "anxiety and depression". He offered some helpful ideas about which brand of anti-depressant and tranquillizer might be most appropriate in her case. She did not take the drugs, but some months later her depression spontaneously lifted and things returned to normal.

Four years later, she was referred again, this time to a psycho-therapist. Her husband had died a few months earlier, at the age of 48, from heart failure. She had been left to run the farm on her own with her 17-year-old adopted son, who was more interested in his motorbike than in helping his mother. She said that she had "coped" very well at first after her husband's death and had "buried herself in the work of getting in the harvest". But when winter came, she felt his absence fully for the first time, and her feelings of panic reappeared.

Her father had died when she was 4 years old, and when her mother remarried she was sent to live with rather Victorian grandparents on a remote farm. She met her husband at 16, and her whole life had revolved around him. He was ill with heart failure for twelve years before his death, and they lived with the knowledge and fear that he might die at any time. Her first episode of anxiety occurred when they decided to sell the dairy herd that they had built up, because he was no longer able to manage the cattle.

During her first session with the psychotherapist, it suddenly struck her that her previous episode of panic had been triggered by the realization, never discussed with her husband, that he was likely to die soon. She cried a little and began to see how cut off she was from her feelings of grief about losing the one significant relationship of her life, and how she had been similarly "cut off in many ways throughout her childhood". After this session she said she felt better and more ready to tackle the farm and her son. The therapist, she said, seemed to "understand how I feel", and she compared this with the previous experience with the psychiatrist, who had asked her "funny questions" and made her wonder if she was going mad.

We have set the stage with this case, unspectacular in itself, because it illustrates some important aspects of the special values of psychotherapy, which forms the subject of this book. Psychotherapy means taking a person seriously. It sees a person all of a piece, a product of her own biography. This understanding, if all goes well, brings relief. It enables the patient to make sense of experiences that were previously incomprehensible, and this in turn enhances the patient's feelings of autonomy and self-esteem. Psychotherapy at this level is not necessarily esoteric or sophisticated, but simply requires listening to patients acutely and trying, collaboratively, to make sense of their experiences.

This case also shows how psychotherapeutic understanding can work at many levels. The first discovery in the session was that the patient's earlier feelings of panic and depression were based on her fears about her husband's illness and subsequent death. A deeper level connected this with her father's ungrieved death and the dependency that characterized her relationship with her husband. Deeper still were fears about her own "mad" upbringing, expressed in her feelings of madness aroused by the psychiatric interview, and the "madness" of her relationship with her adopted son with whom, as with her own mother, she found it so hard to be close. The first psychiatrist "became", in her mind, the grandparents who had failed to understand her; the psychotherapist "became" the husband on whom she had been so dependent, and towards whom she felt guiltily angry for his having died.

The case also illustrates the preventive potential of psychotherapy. It is arguable that, had she (or she and her husband together) had psychotherapy when she first developed symptoms, she (or they) would have been better able to cope with her husband's inevitable death when it came. As well as bringing symptomatic relief, psychotherapy can add strength and depth to the personality so that a person becomes better able to deal with future difficulties.

We see the state of psychotherapy itself as being rather like that of the patient at her previous consultation: it has yet to take itself, or to be taken, seriously. Like the patient who, before therapy, either denies her difficulties or sees them as insuperable, psychotherapy is often blindly supported by its advocates or rejected out of hand by opponents. Neither takes psychotherapy seriously in the sense of seeing it for what it is, both in its strengths and in its weaknesses.

Is psychotherapy worth taking seriously? Does psychotherapy work? Should it become more widely available, especially to the less well-off? Who should be responsible for paying for psychotherapy? What role should psychotherapy play in society? How should consumers be protected against being harmed by exploitative or incompetent therapists? What sort of ethical code or code of practice should govern the conduct of therapists? Should psychotherapy become an organized profession? These are the central questions asked in this book.

What is psychotherapy?

Psychotherapy is enormously diverse. *The Psychotherapy Handbook* (cited in Barker, 1983) lists over 300 types of therapy ranging from Active-Analytic Psychotherapy to Zaraleya Psychoenergetic Technique. Most therapists follow a particular school or tendency, and the authors are no exceptions. Our aim in this book, however, is to consider the whole spectrum of psychotherapy and, as far as possible, to be impartial and non-sectarian. We therefore define psychotherapy in the broadest terms as:

> the systematic use of a relationship between therapist and patient—as opposed to pharmacological or social methods—to produce changes in cognition, feelings, and behaviour.

Our definition would thus include behaviour therapy, family therapy, and psychoanalysis, but exclude drug therapies and electroconvulsive therapy. Despite the apparent diversity of psychotherapies, there are some basic elements that are to be found in all forms of therapy. These may be usefully considered under three headings: *structure, space,* and *relationship* (Holmes, 1986).

Structure

A minimum structure for psychotherapy is an agreed and preferably regular time and place within which therapist and patient can meet. The "visible" structure or form of a session varies greatly between therapies.

Behavioural treatments are usually highly structured. Had the patient we have described been treated with *cognitive behaviour therapy*, she would perhaps have been asked to keep a diary recording her negative thoughts and panicky feelings. She would have been asked to identify recurrent patterns of thought and the assumptions that underlay them. Statements such as "I should be able to be close to my teenage son at all times", or "a 40-year-old farmer's widow is no use to anyone", or "I shall never be able to cope on my own" might have been considered and challenged. The aim of this would have been to lead her to a more realistic and less negative view of herself, and so to be less overwhelmed by fear and grief.

A *family therapist*, on the other hand, might have seen her with her son, and tried to explore their breakdown in communication. Perhaps the boy, by riding his motorbike so fast, was demonstrating his live-liness and determination not to become caught up in his mother's sadness. The mother and son might have been encouraged to talk about their shared loss together.

Gestalt therapy aims to address a person's emotions directly. The patient might have been asked to visualize her husband when he was alive, to "put" him in an "empty chair", and then to try to speak directly to him about her fears and difficulties and her anger and sadness at his loss.

THE ANXIOUS WIDOW (CONTINUED)

In fact the patient was offered "brief analytic therapy" (about twelve sessions), in which there were no pre-determined tasks but she was asked to talk freely about her feelings and fantasies.

She found this difficult and remained inhibited, but attended regularly, and it seemed that therapy was important to her. The therapist had to cancel the sixth session at short notice because he was ill. She in turn missed the following session, but came for the subsequent one in a state of agitation and anger. She had felt very let down by the therapist's absence and felt she could not cope. She reported guiltily that she had been feeling very resentful to-wards her husband for "leaving" her. She began, for the first time in the sessions, to cry uninhibitedly. She said that her present resentment and misery reminded her of loneliness she had experi-enced as a child. This session proved to be a breakthrough, and subsequently she began to look and report feeling much more confident and cheerful. She had managed to go to a family party and enjoy it, but she remained worried about her son.

Although these possible approaches are quite distinct, they have one central feature in common. Each offers a safe structure in which the patient can explore feelings or actions in a controlled way, where the normal consequences of such feelings and actions do not apply. In cognitive behaviour therapy, the patient would be relieved temp-orarily from the responsibilities that made her feel a failure, and so enabled to challenge her negative beliefs about herself. In family therapy, mother and son could row without fear of escalation, and get close without fear of incest. In Gestalt therapy, by speaking to an imaginary husband, the patient would permit herself temporarily to forget the reality of his death. In analytic therapy, the patient could express anger towards the therapist about his absence without feeling that she would have to face retaliation or further loss.

In psychotherapy, as in the theatre, there is a suspension of disbelief, which allows powerful emotions and actions to be explored safely without the consequences that might follow in everyday life. A psychotherapy session, like a play, refers to, reflects on, and is an intensification of reality, but remains, through its formal structure and the neutrality of the therapist, separate from it.

Space

A structure contains. This is important in helping the patient to feel "held" by the treatment, which in itself is a significant therapeutic factor. But the structure does not merely contain: it creates a potential space within which something new can happen. This potential for facilitating self-discovery is another essential feature of psychotherapy. The discovery of new feelings, possibilities, strengths, actions, and attitudes is facilitated by the existence of therapeutic *space*. These discoveries enlarge the patient's self-knowledge and self-esteem. This in turn enhances the ability to cope with, master, or adapt to circumstances. All this fosters the patient's *autonomy*, a concept that we shall return to many times in the course of this book.

There is, however, an apparent paradox within therapy. By entering therapy, a patient appears to be *surrendering* part of her autonomy by accepting the rules and influence of the therapist. Therapy usually has some degree of *regression* built into it, with patients, in the setting of therapy, temporarily becoming more childlike than is normally possible.

There are two reasons why the paradox is merely apparent. First, the dependency that is generated by the therapeutic situation is in the service of greater autonomy in the long run. Within therapy, patients are given a chance to *play*, in the sense of trying out thoughts and actions: in the setting of the therapy, the patient has, like a child, less power, but more liberty. When therapy is successful, the patient develops a sense of inner space and freedom that can be carried over into everyday life.

Second, it needs to be stressed that *autonomy* and *dependency* are not contradictory. Indeed, the capacity to depend and be dependable is an important feature of most successful intimate relationships. Many people seeking psychotherapy suffer from problems concerning dependency. They may feel trapped, and therefore out of control, when they form close relationships; or they may be unable to depend on, and so get close to, others, despite the wish to do so. The opposite of autonomy, therefore, is *not* dependency but *heteronomy*. This means, roughly, "not being in control of one's self". Psychotherapy, often in the setting of secure dependency on a therapist, *reduces* heteronomy by helping the patient to be more aware of, and so less controlled by, experiences and feelings that have been suppressed or ignored. This awareness makes it easier to establish relationships based on mature dependency. In this way, the dependency of the patient on the therapist does not in itself threaten autonomy. (For an extended discussion of autonomy and psychotherapy, see chapter three.)

Despite this, it remains true that some of the ethical dilemmas of psychotherapy do arise out of the cultivation of dependency in the service of increased autonomy.

The therapeutic relationship

The third element, and the most fundamental in psychotherapy, is the therapist–patient relationship. The success of psychotherapy, unlike pharmacotherapy or, say, a correspondence course, depends above all upon the establishment and use of this relationship to produce change. This is not to say that drug treatments and correspondence courses do *not* depend upon human interactions that are also relevant to their efficacy. But, in psychotherapy, the relationship with the therapist is the main instrument of treatment.

In this book we shall be particularly concerned with the ethical implications of the therapist–patient relationship. Since the nature of the therapeutic relationship varies greatly from therapy to therapy, so too do the ethical dilemmas.

In behaviour therapy, the therapist usually adopts the role of teacher, motivator, and director. The therapist instructs the patient what to do, how to overcome fears and failures, how to change irrational attitudes and beliefs. In this type of treatment, the relationship between patient and therapist is not unlike that between traditional teacher and pupil. One ethical danger is that the therapist may be tempted to abuse this position, becoming coercive rather than therapeutic.

By contrast, in analytic psychotherapy encouragement is implicit rather than overt. Patients have usually already been given advice by well-meaning friends and relations. They enter therapy in search of emotional freedom and understanding and seeking a special intimacy with the therapist, one that is perhaps unique to psychotherapeutic relationships. It depends on a focused but non-controlling attention on the part of the therapist. Therapists must listen empathically without the need to intrude. The therapist's job is to help patients discover and clarify their own feelings, not to guide, advise, direct, or pity. All this places the therapist in a position of considerable responsibility, different from other professions; for the patient is entrusting not her bank balance, the roof of her house, or even her malfunctioning body, but her very self. The therapist is guardian of feelings, fears, and fantasies which the patient may never have revealed to anyone before, not even herself. The ethical responsibilities this imposes need special consideration and discussion.

A central ethical issue for psychotherapy follows from the fact that therapists are in a position of relative power, while patients seeking therapy are often in a weak state, in desperate search for an answer to their problems. The more powerful the therapist's personal qualities and therapeutic ideology, the more the patient may be attracted to the therapist. Although this power is useful in creating a positive attitude on the part of the patient, it can also be dangerous. Patients may become so dependent on the therapist that their autonomy really is put at risk. Although such dependency may be better than what preceded it, there is always the danger that therapeutic dependency may provide opportunities that bad therapists can exploit. Financial and sexual abuse of patients by therapists undoubtedly occur, and we shall consider what safeguards are needed to minimize them.

Psychoanalytic therapy attempts, through the concept of *transference*, to make the issue of dependency-in-the-service-of-autonomy a central vehicle for therapeutic change. When one of Freud's early patients, "Anna O", threw her arms around his neck in a passionate embrace, he did not, like his colleague Breuer, quickly retreat into the safer streams of conventional medicine, nor did he thank his luck and enjoy the situation (Freud, 1895d). He tried instead to understand what was happening. He maintained that the feelings aroused in his patients were not an appreciation of his own irresistible charms, but belonged to a quite different context—that of daughter and father. These feelings had been *transferred* onto the person of the therapist just as, in our example, the farmer's wife transferred her feelings about her grandparents and husband onto the psychiatrist and psychotherapist respectively. If the patient could become aware of her feelings, she would be on the way to a cure: no longer would she be in the grip of the past, but she would be able to see her actions and feelings for what they were. Through the arousal and analysis of transference, psychoanalytic therapy aims to evoke feelings of dependency, but to use them so as to enhance the patient's autonomy. This may be compared with the Brechtian theory of theatre: the audience has to be enthralled, but also to be reminded of the artifice that has evoked their thraldom. In this way, theatre becomes an agent of change and widened freedom, capable of moving the audience to see their lives and environment more clearly, rather than merely being an anodyne escape from immutable miseries.

Classification of therapies

So far we have described some common elements in various types of psychotherapy. How, then, should we classify the different forms of therapy? As with religious or political sects, these differences, so vital-seeming to their adherents, can seem obscure to the public.

Despite their diversity, psychotherapies can be grouped together into a fairly small number of categories, according to their theoretical orientation and founders. These include the *analytic therapies* derived from Freud and Jung; *client-centred therapies* derived from Carl Rogers; *humanistic or active therapies* such as bioenergetics, Gestalt, and psychodrama, started respectively by Wilhelm Reich, Fritz Perls, and Jacob Moreno; *family therapies* based on systems theory derived from the ideas of Gregory Bateson; and *behavioural* and *cognitive therapies* associated with J. Watson, S. Wolpe, and George Kelly (see Glossary).

These different theoretical orientations can also be classified according to what goes on in the therapy sessions. *Directive* therapies (behaviour therapy and some types of family therapy) emphasize overt behaviour rather than experience, and therapists often issue precise instructions and directions to their patients. The basis of *reflec-*

tive therapies (analytic and client-centred) is the Wordsworthian concept of "emotion recollected in tranquillity". By holding up a mirror to the patient's actions and feelings, therapy enables them to be seen for what they are, to be understood, and where necessary to be changed. *Expressive* therapies (active therapies) aim to help with emotional self-expression by directly evoking emotional and bodily feelings in therapy sessions.

The attempt to classify therapies is complicated by three factors. First, most contain, in varying amounts, a combination of expression, direction, and reflection; second, what therapists do in sessions is often different from what they say or think they do; and third, most therapies are not static but evolving, and are more commonly hybrids than pure forms.

The convergence of the psychotherapies while retaining their separate identities is, in our view, one of the positive features of contemporary psychotherapy. The recent development of cognitive behavioural therapies, for example, means that behaviour therapists now recognize the inner world of their patients and are beginning to build bridges with analytic therapies (Ryle, 1982). These therapies attempt to change not just patients' external behaviour, but also their mental structures and attitudes.

At the same time, recent developments in psychoanalytic therapy, especially the emergence of brief analytic therapies, mean that many analytic therapists are much more than merely reflective, actively encouraging their patients to think about certain aspects of their lives, and pushing them to express feelings towards the therapist more clearly and openly. This is perhaps no more than a return to some of Freud's methods. He often pressed his interpretations on his patients forcefully (and would reward himself with a cigar if the patient accepted them!) (Roazen, 1979).

Expressive therapies usually have a dramatic quality to them, and they too draw on one of Freud's earliest ideas: that neurosis is caused by trauma which, if relived in therapy, can be relieved by catharsis. Neurosis is now thought to be more a product of cumulative rather than single trauma, and catharsis a rare phenomenon, which many therapists would view with suspicion. Nevertheless, active techniques can be a valuable way of helping patients to break through intellectual defences and so experience emotions rather than just talking about them.

Sometimes the type of therapy refers not to its *mode* or approach, but rather to the *arrangements* under which it is conducted. For example, individual, family, or group therapy may each be analytic, behavioural, or humanistic.

Another important dimension is the *length* of therapy. Prolonged therapies are particularly associated with psychoanalysis, which typically consists of three to five sessions per week over several years, and is virtually only available in the private sector. In some patients, this degree of intensity may be needed to produce lasting change. The investment of time involved raises questions for publicly funded treatment, which we shall discuss. If psychotherapy is to be taken seriously, is it legitimate to have a two-tier system—with prolonged therapy available only to those who can afford it and who happen to live in those parts of the country where it is available, while brief therapy is usually the only treatment to be offered through public funding?

The role of the therapist constitutes another dimension along which therapies vary. Psychotherapy has been described as the "purchase of friendship" (Schofield, 1965). But in therapy, typically only the patient is self-revealing, unlike the mutual self-revelation of friendship. Patients often complain of this, and the extent to which therapy and friendship should or should not overlap is one of the points of conflict between "fringe" therapies and more orthodox treatment. This, too, requires discussion and may need to form part of a code of practice of psychotherapists. For some, the curative aspect of therapy is the "unconditional positive regard" or love offered by the therapist to patients. For others it is their technical skill. In practice, both are necessary, but it must always be remembered that at the root of any therapy there lies a human encounter.

Psychotherapists and their training

We have discussed the variety of psychotherapies. But who are the psychotherapists and how do they become what they are? The public tend to be confused by the terms "psychiatrist", "psychologist", "psychotherapist", and "psychoanalyst", and we have tried to clarify the distinctions between them in the Glossary.

Although the original psychoanalysts were almost all medically trained, Freud was a passionate advocate of "lay" analysis. Psychotherapists today may be doctors, clinical psychologists, social workers, priests, marriage guidance counsellors, or indeed lack any formal qualifications, either in psychotherapy or in any other profession. At present, in the United Kingdom it is not illegal for anyone who chooses to do so to call herself a psychotherapist. As with a poet or a window cleaner, the activity itself justifies the title. University degrees courses in psychotherapy (almost all at postgraduate level) are becoming more widespread, but most are in psychoanalytic theory and do not equip the student to be a practicing psychotherapist. This in itself is not necessarily a bad thing. Some, although surprisingly few, of our best poets have not studied literature at university. The existence of a profession does not in itself guarantee a good service to the public. In some fields, standardized training may mean mediocrity and uniformity in an area that, because of the variety of human situations, calls out for diversity. But, as far as we know, a bad poem never did any harm, and the results of a bad or rude window cleaner are immediately visible and easy to put right. Psychotherapy, on the other hand, *can* do harm, either positively by making patients worse, or negatively by not producing significant change; and these results may only appear after considerable time, money, and emotional effort have been expended. The need for some regulation of psychotherapy training has therefore become apparent: the form it should take is still an area of active debate.

Members of the "core professions"—psychiatry, psychology, social work, nursing—learn psychotherapy as part of their training, but the psychotherapeutic content of this training may be patchy, superficial, or one-sided. The vast majority of psychotherapists have trained in the private sector. Almost all reputable psychotherapy training organizations are now affiliated to an "umbrella" organization, The United Kingdom Council for Psychotherapy (UKCP). A number of psychoanalytically oriented trainings have formed the British Confederation of Psychothapists (BCP). Trainings vary considerably in the length, depth, and costs of their training and in the stringency of their entry requirements. Psychoanalytic training, for example, requires a medical or other good university degree and relevant experience in the helping professions as an entry requirement, together with a searching assessment of the candidate's maturity and capacity for development. The course lasts for about four years and consists of personal analysis, at least two cases treated under supervision, and a series of theoretical seminars. The process is, for many, prohibitively expensive. On the other hand, there are several organizations that offer shorter and cheaper training courses, producing psychotherapists who, some would argue, are no less good. Psychoanalysts justify their training on the grounds that they can treat more serious cases (although there is no definite evidence that they do) and are in a position to teach on the less rigorous training courses. If, as we believe it should, psychotherapy becomes recognized as a profession, and more public funding becomes available for both training and treatment, these issues, and the assumptions that underlie them, will have to be disentangled and confronted.

Another important issue about training is whether or not psychotherapists should have their own personal therapy. At present, it is only analytic therapists who insist on this, and behaviour therapists are, on the whole, opposed to the idea, although some now accept that personal support, say in a group, can be very helpful. The argument turns partly on the nature of psychotherapy as a discipline. In our view, although analogous in some respects to education and medicine, psychotherapy has many features that make it unique. As far as training is concerned it can perhaps be usefully compared with child-rearing: just as the best preparation for parenthood is to have had a successful upbringing oneself, so the internalization of a good personal therapeutic experience can be one—but perhaps not the only—route to the self-awareness and maturity that are needed to be a good psychotherapist.

Psychotherapy and its critics

Opposition to psychotherapy, and in particular to psychoanalysis, has always been fierce. Freud, in his early days, was virtually ostracized by his medical colleagues because of his insistence on the importance of sexuality in the origin of neurosis. Although the grounds have shifted from morality to science and politics, the opposition is no less fierce today.

Critics like Karl Popper, Peter Medawar, Ernest Gellner, and Hans Eysenck object to the apparent lack of scientific rigour that underlies most psychotherapeutic theories. They portray psychoanalysis and many psychotherapies as latter-day religions masquerading as science, immune to criticism or falsifiability, offering false hope to those in distress, lead balloons destined for well-deserved extinction. There may be some substance in these charges, especially when applied to the quasi-mystical fringes of psychotherapy. But our concern in this book is with psychotherapy as a whole, and we show in chapter two that there is now strong evidence for the effectiveness of psychotherapy. More importantly, we argue that such criticism ultimately fails to grasp and take seriously the central contributions of psychoanalysis and psychotherapy to modern thought. These include an insistence on the importance of the inner world; the reality of unconscious motivation; the vital role of the imagination, as well as reason; the part played by childhood experience in moulding character and relationships in adult life; the influence of these relationships on feelings and behaviour; and, above all, the capacity of therapy to enhance maturation and autonomy. We argue that the outright rejection of psychotherapy as "unscientific" is, in any case, unjustified and arises from a narrow *scientism*, rather than from sound principles of philosophy of science.

Psychotherapy has also been the subject of political critique. We argue that psychotherapy addresses fundamental needs for emotional autonomy, satisfying relationships, and self-esteem and that it should therefore be regarded as part of essential care, and become much more widely available. But even among those who appreciate the value of psychotherapy, its expansion is often viewed with suspicion—by critics at opposite ends of the political spectrum.

On the one hand, there are those who fear that psychotherapy may be used essentially as a palliative, diverting attention away from the true cause of human unhappiness—which in their view is a society divided by class, racism, and sexism (Epstein, 1995). Psychotherapy is no solution, they claim, and indeed may constitute a further degradation or mystification, moulding people so that they find the truly intolerable tolerable.

On the other hand, right-wing libertarians such as the psychoanalyst Thomas Szasz argue that although the poor may have material needs, they do not need psychotherapy; that state-funded institutions serve the interests of the state rather than the individual; and that if there is to be psychotherapy, it should therefore be available only to those able and willing to pay for it under a private contract with their therapists.

We shall argue that each of these claims, although containing a grain of truth, is mistaken. Useful analogies can be drawn with state-funded education, which has been criticized from both extremes of the political spectrum as an instrument of social control. Such allegations do have *some* plausibility. However, education is a precondition both for the "autonomous individuality" celebrated by libertarians, and for the "true revolutionary class consciousness" required by Marxism. We shall argue that, far from being a diversion or a luxury, psychotherapy, like education, may well be essential in a modern industrial society, and that the solution to the problem of it being used for doubtful purposes is to insist on proper controls, rather than to oppose its expansion.

Psychotherapy, as we see it, has a specific ideological contribution to make in modern society. It restores the inner, private world of the individual and his family to what Habermas calls the "public sphere" (cited in Eagleton, 1985). By this is not meant the street corner or the hustings, but an arena of social reality, subject to change, open to analysis and discussion. The feminist movement, which undoubtedly has psychotherapeutic roots, however critical it may be of the chauvinistic aspects of therapy, is an example of a social force that has brought a particular segment of "private" life into the realm of public debate. Similarly, psychotherapy, both in its private encounter with the patient and in its public face, has responsibility for a part of human experience that, in our society, only it takes seriously. Our aim in this book is, by taking psychotherapy seriously, to help with this task.

Psychotherapy as essential care

Psychotherapy, which in its modern form has one of its most significant roots in Freudian psychoanalysis, is now firmly established in the public imagination and is beginning, slowly, to achieve recognition among the professions. In Britain, for example, psychiatrists, many of whom have hitherto been ambivalent about or even implacably opposed to psychoanalysis, now insist that all psychiatrists receive some exposure to psychotherapy as part of their training. Modern scientific medicine has rediscovered the importance of the doctor–patient relationship and is turning its attention to the uses of psychotherapy in stress reduction and healing. Psychology is no longer exclusively concerned with behavioural science, and it now seeks a much wider brief. The influence of psychotherapy can be found throughout the education system, from pre-school playgroups to universities. Psychoanalytic ideas are now firmly established in parts of the academic world, especially in anthropology, literature, sociology, and linguistics. Social policy, notably in the areas of child-care and the penal system, is also influenced by psychoanalytic thought. In general, psychotherapy has become a tangible presence which cannot be ignored.

Nevertheless, although psychotherapy has a presence, it has yet to find a secure home. There are important issues to be resolved about psychotherapy as a theory, as a practical method of treatment, and as a profession, many of which we discuss in the course of this book.

The efficacy of psychotherapy is an active area of discussion and conflict. Wild claims and hopes have been expressed for its universal applicability as a treatment for all mental disorders, while opponents argue that it is of no value at all. What are the ways in which psycho-therapy can, and cannot, help people?

The polarization of opinion about the value of psychotherapy is reflected in its uneven availability and distribution. In the United Kingdom, for instance, London and a few urban centres have consid-erable psychotherapy resources, while some regions of the country have virtually none. There is a similar bias in the distribution of psychotherapy by social class. Psychotherapy is beyond the reach, pocket, and ken of many poorer patients who could well benefit from it. At present psychotherapy is both ideologically and practically the provenance of a certain fairly narrow class section of the population. Should steps be taken to foster awareness of psychotherapy and to make it much more widely available, even at a (fairly modest, we shall argue) cost to the ubiquitous taxpayer?

A third area where psychotherapy has yet to find its home centres on its status as a profession. We have already mentioned the need for regulation and supervision of psychotherapy training. There is a similar need for scrutiny of ethical and technical standards of practice, a task that the UKCP has set out to fulfil. The impact of the UKCP (which has been in existence for less than a decade) is only just beginning to be felt. The content and quality of what is called "psychotherapy" remains enormously variable, The UKCP and BCP publish lists of therapists who are members of accredited training organizations, which offers the public some protection, but quality-control of trainings is still embryonic and choice of therapist remains fairly random, despite the evidence that matching of a client's problem to appropriate therapy is likely to produce a better outcome than the current system of chance encounter and personal recommendation (Roth & Fonagy, 1996). This position, as Jonathan Pedder (1988) has pointed out, is not unlike that of the medical profession in the first half of the nineteenth century at the time when statutory regulation of medical training and practice was being established. The formation of a state-recognized, -regulated, and -registered psychotherapy profession would go some way to improving standards of training, technique, and ethics. We are strongly in favour of this, but wide discussion continues to be needed if a structure and organization for psychotherapy is to be found that can meet public need and, at the same time, avoid the pitfalls of protectionism and self-interest to which the professions are liable.

In the first half of the book we present a philosophical, ethical, technical, economic, and political case for seeking a wide expansion of publicly funded psychotherapy.

If psychotherapy *is* to be expanded, the ethical and other practical questions we have mentioned will assume a pressing urgency. What are the special moral responsibilities of a psychotherapist? How should therapists balance their concern for their patients with responsibilities to the wider community? How can the public best be protected against the risk of exploitation and abuse by unscrupulous therapists? Should the state begin to regulate the psychotherapy profession, and if so, how? We consider these issues in the second half of the book.

Our immediate task is to answer the case against psychotherapy. This we begin in the next chapter.

CHAPTER TWO

The case
against psychotherapy

One of the most important claims of this book is that psychotherapy should become much more widely available; indeed that it should be regarded as no less essential than
other forms of health care, or education. We argue this case in detail
in chapters three and four. But, if this ambitious claim is to be worthy
of serious consideration, it is necessary first to answer several criticisms of psychotherapy, the most serious of which are: that psychotherapy is unscientific; that it does not work, even on its own terms;
and that even when it does work, it does not offer its beneficiaries
anything worth the expense. We attempt to answer these criticisms
in this and the next chapter. A final criticism concerns the social role
of psychotherapy, and whether it is, or could be, a disguised tool of
social control. This is considered further in chapter five.

We start with the questions of scientific status and efficacy because, unless psychotherapy can offer a reasonable answer to them,
our moral argument for more resources to be put into psychotherapy
would, at best, be of merely academic interest—for there could be
no justification in seeking public support for a practice that is ill-
founded and of little benefit.

There is a wealth of literature on the scientific status (Taylor, 1987) and efficacy (Garfield & Bergin, 1986) of psychotherapy (see Roth & Fonagy, 1996, for an up-to-date and authoritative summary), and it would be inappropriate for a book of this sort to try to offer a detailed or definitive analysis of this research. Our aim in this chapter is merely to defuse some of the more damaging charges that have been laid against psychotherapy. Our intent is to clear the ground for the subsequent discussion of the case for regarding psychotherapy as a part of essential care, and as a proper subject for serious ethical consideration.

In considering the scientific status of psychotherapy, we immediately encounter a number of difficulties. First, there is the variety of psychotherapies. Most philosophical discussion of the scientific status of psychotherapy has been directed towards psychoanalysis, partly in response to Freud's insistence that psychoanalysis be considered a science. The scientific claims of behavioural therapies have gone almost without challenge, while the more humanistic therapies have themselves been ambivalent about whether they wish to be accorded scientific status. In this book, we consider the entire spectrum of psychotherapies, but in the first part of this chapter we confine ourselves to psychoanalysis since, of all forms of psychotherapy, this is the one that has most often been accused of being unscientific.

The second difficulty is that scientific evaluation of psychotherapy can take many forms. Philosophical criticism has tended to focus on the question of whether psychotherapy is *in principle* capable of scientific evaluation by asking such questions as: "Are the propositions of psychoanalytic theory falsifiable?" Much of this debate is, to the practising psychotherapist, scholastic in tone and far removed from clinical reality. Many of the general propositions of psychoanalysis—for example the tenet that the liability to adult psychological disorder is strongly influenced by childhood experience—are well established (Bowlby, 1988), while some of the more doubtful assertions of classical psychoanalysis—for example, that all dreams invariably represent disguised wishes—are now regarded by most clinicians as mistaken. Clinicians tend to be less interested in philosophical questions about the scientific status of their particular theories than with the evaluation of psychotherapy as a *treatment*. Can psychotherapy help people to recover from psychological illness or distress, and, if so, how does this come about? These questions are discussed in the second part of the chapter.

Is psychoanalysis scientific?

The ultimate criterion of whether or not a theory is scientific is its testability. But what constitutes testability has become controversial. It used to be held that testability required confirmation by facts. To adopt this criterion could, however, produce the embarrassing consequence that no empirical theory is truly scientific. For, as Karl Popper, echoing Hume, pointed out, no finite number of observations of a correlation entails that the correlation will hold in hitherto unobserved cases (Popper, 1960). This recognition led Popper to propose *falsifiability* as the test of a scientific theory.

A common objection raised against psychoanalysis is that it is unfalsifiable. According to this criticism in its simplest form, because psychoanalytic theory purports to explain everything about the mental world, it really explains nothing. No evidence could show that psychoanalytic theory is false, since any psychological observation would be consistent with the theory. The theory is therefore vacuous and cannot form the basis of serious scientific research.

One of the cornerstones of psychoanalytic theory is the theory of the unconscious. This claims that, in the explanation of human motivation, conscious experience forms but the tip of an iceberg; conscious thoughts and feelings rest on a base of unconscious thoughts and impulses, some of which are actively kept out of awareness by repression and other defence mechanisms. What could count as evidence against such a claim? One would apparently need to produce cases of conscious motivation in which unconscious forces play no part. But, so the argument goes, such a case could never be produced. Suppose that in a particular case no unconscious motivation could be detected. This would still not be evidence that such motivation was *absent*, since unconscious forces, by their very nature, cannot be observed. So psychoanalytic theory is unscientific, because it cannot be tested.

There are two issues here: first, the general objection that no observation *could* count against the thesis that there is such a thing as unconscious motivation; second, the claim that the specific hypotheses of psychoanalysis are in principle unfalsifiable. Let us consider them in turn.

It is true that no single observation could count as evidence against the fundamental claim that there is unconscious motivation. But this in itself does not undermine the scientific status of psychoanalysis. Uncontroversially scientific theories such as those of Newtonian physics rest on axioms that are presupposed by the theory. Newton assumed the truth of Galileo's Principle of Inertia, for example, according to which bodies will continue in motion in a straight line unless acted on by an external force; and this cannot be refuted by the observation of a body that deviates from a straight line despite not apparently being acted on by any external force. When a Newtonian observes a body changing direction, he looks for the external force, even if it cannot be detected immediately. A psychoanalyst looks for unconscious motivation in a similar way.

These fundamental assumptions or axioms are clearly not subject to piecemeal falsification through observation: their role as axioms excludes this. The crucial question is whether or not the axioms, when combined with other plausible assumptions and observations, yield useful or interesting predictions and explanations. The fact that the fundamental assumption of the primacy of unconscious forces is not directly falsifiable by any single observed counter-example does not in itself tell against psychoanalytic theory.

The second objection is of more concern. Within normal natural science, where it is claimed that there is a link between two phenomena, the two phenomena can each be observed—as, for example, with the claim that the presence of an extra chromosome causes Down's syndrome. The apparent problem with psychoanalysis is that when it is claimed that there is a connection between a current psychological condition and the presence of unconscious motives, the unconscious motives cannot be directly observed, so it is impossible to construct determinate experiments to test such claims. Therefore, so the argument goes, it is impossible for any observation to falsify a specific psychoanalytic hypothesis. Therefore psychoanalysis is unscientific.

There are four responses to this objection. First, contrary to the argument, certain specific psychoanalytic hypotheses *have* been refuted—at least to the satisfaction of the majority of psychoanalysts. For example, it used to be held by psychoanalysts that paranoia was caused by repressed homosexuality. This is now regarded as oversimplistic, or even just plain false. Analysts would regard it as incompatible with the clinical observation that not all the paranoid *are* repressed homosexuals.

Second, while it is true that individual unconscious psychological states cannot be directly observed but must be inferred from behaviour, including verbal behaviour, this does not mean that there can be no evidence for their presence in particular situations. Most of our ordinary knowledge about *conscious* psychological states is inferential; and all scientific observations are relative to a set of theoretical assumptions as to what is to count as evidence for the phenomenon in question. A psychoanalyst may legitimately infer the likelihood of repressed homosexual feelings from dreams, slips of the tongue, and the patient's behaviour in the transference.

A third line of defence is to point out that it is unreasonable to expect a psychological theory to conform to the same strict principles of measurement that apply to the natural sciences. Donald Davidson has argued, in a way that has commanded widespread acceptance among philosophers, that there can be no strict psychological laws (Davidson, 1980). A *psychological* explanation of an agent's behaviour aims to show how it is *reasonable* or rationally intelligible in the light of that agent's beliefs and desires. Because an individual's beliefs and desires do not exist as atoms in isolation from one another, it is not possible to produce exceptionless laws relating the presence of a particular belief-type to a certain kind of behaviour. On this view, if Freud or anyone else was attempting to produce a strictly scientific psychology, they would inevitably fail. In this respect psychoanalytic theory is no worse off than any other psychological theory, and the fact that no theory can generate interesting exceptionless psychological laws is not a reason for abandoning psychology.

Finally, it should be pointed out that the psychoanalytic theory of the unconscious is in effect an extension of common-sense belief–desire psychology. Our common-sense belief–desire psychology offers the best method currently available for predicting how people are likely to behave, and in most situations it is adequate to the task. Furthermore, and quite apart from the question of prediction, human beings are, and perhaps always will be, concerned to understand and explain their own and other people's behaviour by reference to their beliefs and desires. Unless one assumes that there are unconscious psychological states, much of our behaviour will be rationally unintelligible. With the supposition that they do exist, many gaps can be filled. To illustrate this, let us consider the following example.

THE ANGRY COLLEAGUE

A man, whose father was dying of lung cancer, began to have violent rows with a female colleague at work about her lack of diligence and poor time-keeping. He had not argued with her before, and was surprised and upset by his, on the whole, counter-productive outbursts, which were uncharacteristic and out of all proportion to the situation. His behaviour during this time remained a mystery until, some time later, during psycho-analysis, he realized that unconsciously he had displaced and projected many of the feelings associated with his father's ill-ness—rage and anger, disappointment in the doctors whom he felt had been less than diligent, sadness about the lack of time left for his father, childlike disappointment in his mother for failing to keep her husband alive—onto the female colleague. For the first time he had an intelligible explanation of what had been inexplic-able behaviour.

A sceptic might ask: "What evidence do you have that this is a genuine explanation, rather than simply a psychoanalytic interpreta-tion without foundation?" The evidence is likely to be complex, including, for example, appeal to the well-documented finding that bottling-up grief leads to increased anxiety, which leads to irascibil-ity; the fact that the purported discovery was accompanied by a sense of relief in the man; and the fact that projection and displacement are well-established psychological and (in the case of displacement) etho-logical phenomena that can be observed in many other clinical and non-clinical situations. It should be noted that although some of this evidence itself uses psychoanalytic concepts, this is no more an objec-tion to it than it would be an objection to research in quantum physics that quantum concepts figure in its explanations.

Although the evidence is complex and may always be subject to possible revision in the light of future discoveries, this does not mean it should carry no rational persuasion. It is really no more than an extension of ordinary explanations in terms of *conscious* beliefs and desires. As we have argued, they are not directly observed either.

Is psychoanalysis a pseudo-science?

Even if psychoanalytic theory is in principle subject to some kind of testing, a worry is sometimes expressed by critics that its practition-ers, particularly Freud, have systematically resisted putting it to the test. Two philosophers who have written extensively about this are Cioffi (1970) and Grunbaum (1984). In his controversial paper "Freud and the Idea of a Pseudo-Science" (1970), Cioffi claims that psychoanalysis is not a genuine empirical enterprise. He likens psychoanalysis to other "pseudo-diagnostic, pseudo-therapeutic or pseudo-explanatory claims", among which he includes astrology, numerology, and phrenology. He writes:

> ... to establish that an enterprise is pseudo-scientific it is not sufficient to show that the procedures it employs would *in fact* prevent or obstruct the discovery of disconfirmatory states of affairs but that it is their function to obstruct such discovery. To claim that an enterprise is pseudo-scientific is to claim that it involves the habitual and wilful employment of methodologically defective procedures (in a sense of wilful which encompasses refined self-deception). [Cioffi, 1970]

Psychoanalytic theory assumes that adverse early childhood relationships and bodily emotional experience play an important part in creating vulnerability to psychological breakdown in the face of stress in adult life. The psychoanalyst seeks to find links between the patient's current psychological state and earlier experience. The relevant memories of the past, especially childhood, are often inaccessible. Therapy therefore aims, through analysis of transference, dreams, and free association, to provide a method for recalling this information in order to enable the patient to understand the forces that drive her to behave and feel the way she does. The analyst works by offering *interpretations* of what her patient says. These link a current difficulty, transference feelings towards the analyst, and early childhood experience, trying to find a pattern common to all three. An important test of the truth or otherwise of such an interpretation is the patient's response to it, both verbal and non-verbal.

But on Cioffi's view, the psychoanalyst is put in a position in which she becomes insulated from, rather than seeks, the truth. Suppose the analyst puts forward an interpretation that is strongly *resisted* by the patient. This may be taken by the analyst as evidence that the interpretation is on the right lines (according to the Queen Gertrude principle: "Methinks the lady doth protest too much"), and is encountering the patient's defence mechanisms. Cioffi's objection is that psychoanalytic theory is so constructed as to make it unlikely that the analyst will accept the possibility that the patient is angry because the patient thinks *correctly* that the interpretation is outrageously off-beam. What if the patient agrees with the interpretation? This, too, would not *establish* its truth, since psychoanalytic theory might itself predict that patients would produce material likely to be pleasing to psychoanalysts, as part of "positive transference". If a patient stubbornly refuses to accept interpretations this, on the other hand, could be part of "negative transference" (for a detailed discussion of ethical problems raised by transference, see chapter six).

An explanation on psychoanalytic lines of the patient mentioned at the start of chapter one might go as follows:

THE ANXIOUS WIDOW (CONTINUED)

The patient was, partly as a result of her childhood bereavement and separation from her mother, very dependent on her husband. She had few inner resources and, as happens in many marriages, used her husband as an "auxiliary ego" on whom she relied for strength. A more straightforward psychology than psychoanalysis might have predicted that when he died she would become inconsolably grief-stricken. In fact, she carried on almost as though nothing had happened. She was unable to mourn, and when things did begin to go wrong it was anxiety she experienced, not sadness. She defended herself against internal collapse by at first feeling nothing, and later worrying unduly about minor matters. Her feelings of grief, anger, and despair remained unconscious.

Critics claim that this kind of account puts the therapists in a position where they are always right. If the farmer's wife becomes inconsolably grief-stricken, that supports the hypothesis of weak internal ego; if she feels nothing, that *equally* supports the theory. Let us call such explanations "explanations in the alternative". It seems that the battery of concepts used by psychoanalysis and its psychotherapeutic descendants lend themselves to insulation from hard confrontation with the facts. Cioffi is especially critical of the use of explanations in the alternative, and attempts to ridicule Freud's use of them, taking the example of Freud's claim that there is a significant relationship between the strictness of a person's father and the development of an over-strict superego (and thus a tendency to suffer from guilt feelings). He uses the following two quotations from (different parts of) Freud's work:

> If the father was hard, violent and cruel, the super-ego takes over these attributes from him, and in the relations between the ego and it, the passivity which was supposed to have been repressed is re-established. The super-ego has become sadistic, and the ego becomes masochistic. . . . A great need for punishment develops within the ego, which in part offers itself as a victim to fate, and in part finds satisfaction in ill-treatment by the super-ego (that is, the sense of guilt). [Freud, 1950]

> The unduly lenient and indulgent father fosters the development of an over-strict super-ego because, in the face of the love which is showered on it, the child has no other way of disposing of its aggressiveness than to turn it inwards. [Freud, 1930a]

Cioffi concludes:

> That is, if a child develops a sadistic super-ego, either he had a harsh and punitive father or he had not. But this is just what we might expect if there were no relation between his father's character and the harshness of his super-ego. [Cioffi, 1970]

Cioffi's inference from the two passages is certainly unwarranted (Cosin, Freeman, & Freeman, 1972). The first passage points out how a sadistic superego can be the product of *over-harsh* parenting by the father. The second describes how *over-indulgent* parenting can also lead to "an over-strict super-ego". Cioffi infers that this implies there is *no* connection between relations with one's father and the severity of the superego. However, it is not difficult to see that the two accounts are equally consistent with the more plausible view that *both* over-indulgent *and* over-severe fathering are likely to produce a pathological sense of guilt, and that a good father has to steer, in Aristotelian fashion, a middle course between indulgence and severity.

It is undoubtedly true that psychoanalysis *can* be, and sometimes is, misused in the way Cioffi is concerned about. Indeed, as we argue in the second half of this book, it is this very possibility that creates the need for stringent technical and ethical standards in psychotherapy. But it does not follow from this that psychoanalysis is always used in this way, still less that it *has* to be. A defender of psychoanalysis would claim that the explanations in the alternative which Cioffi criticizes are necessary because of the material with which they are dealing. If it is true, as most would concede, that human motivation is complex, in that individuals are subject to conflicting desires and have conflicting reasons for action, then any simple explanation is unlikely to be true.

No doubt it is *sometimes* true that the patient is resisting the correct interpretation of her actions; sometimes the explanation that the patient seems keen to accept is *not* true; sometimes actions are over-determined, having more than one explanation. It is therefore part of the complexity of psychological life, as revealed by psychoanalysis, that one cannot always accept people's adamant denial of an interpretation. On the other hand, it is equally true, as many would be the first to admit, that therapists often get things wrong. The key issue concerns the nature of psychoanalytic evidence, or what constitutes a psychoanalytic "fact" (see Tuckett, 1995). Grunbaum is much less sceptical than Cioffi about the scientific status of psychoanalysis, which he sees as having empirical *potential*, much of which has yet to be realized. He bases his case on Freud's "tally" argument based on the idea that when an interpretation given by the analyst tallies with the patient's experience, there will be an emotional response which is in itself evidence of the accuracy or otherwise of the interpretation. This approach has been exploited in psychotherapy process research (Shapiro, 1995).

Because of the complexity of psychological life, and because the material that is the subject-matter of psychoanalytic enquiry consists of memories that have usually been buried and hidden, evidence may be conflicting, and the enquiry is inevitably difficult and subject to error. This does mean that unscrupulous or inexperienced analysts may exploit these uncertainties in order to preserve their own cherished beliefs, or to promote some other unworthy purpose. The fact that this makes psychoanalysis open to abuse does not, however, mean that such abuse is intrinsic to it. The fact that fundamentalist Christian geologists said that fossils were deposited simultaneously in different layers of the earth's substratum in order to test people's faith in God does not cast doubt on the authenticity of *geology*. What is crucial to both geology and psychoanalysis is that they are, and should remain, dynamic disciplines whose theories adapt to new observations and theories.

Resistances to psychoanalysis?

One of the difficulties attendant on evaluating the arguments over the validity of psychoanalytic theory is that the protagonists are very suspicious of each other's motives. Thus Cioffi more or less accuses

Freud of being a fraud, and much of his argument supposedly against *psychoanalysis* rests on such an assumption. Webster (1996) has similarly suggested that Freud systematically concealed the true facts of his cases in order to make them appear in a more favourable light.

The title of Freud's paper "Resistances to Psychoanalysis" (1925e) implies that he regarded many objections to his theories as psychological rather than logical. In therapy, individuals have to overcome their resistance and defences against their inner feelings and face the truth about themselves, however uncomfortable or disequilibrating that process may be. Objections to psychoanalysis, Freud suggests, may consist not just of reasoned arguments against it, but also of resistance to a view of human nature and a practice of psychiatry that threatens existing values. This is how he characterizes the medical profession's opposition to psychoanalysis:

> Doctors regard it as a speculative system and refuse to believe that, like every other natural science, it is based on patient and tireless elaboration of facts from the world of perception. . . . They had been brought up to respect only anatomical, physical and chemical factors. They were not prepared for taking psychical ones into account, and therefore met them with indifference or antipathy. They obviously had doubts whether psychical events allowed of any exact scientific treatment whatever. . . . They regarded such abstractions as those with which psychology is obliged to work as nebulous, fantastic and mystical; while they simply refused to believe in remarkable phenomena which might have been the starting-point of research. The symptoms of hysterical neurosis were looked upon as shamming, and the phenomena of hypnotism as a hoax. Even the psychiatrists, upon whose attention the most unusual and astonishing mental phenomena were constantly being forced, showed no inclination to examine their details or enquire into their connections. They were content to classify the variegated array of symptoms and trace them back, so far as they could manage, to somatic, anatomical or chemical aetiological disturbances. During this materialistic, or rather mechanistic period, medicine made tremendous advances, but it also showed a short-sighted misunderstanding of the most important and most difficult among the problems of life. [Freud, 1925e]

Relations between psychoanalysis and the medical establishment have continued to be uneasy, and the debate has continued. In comparison with some contemporary attacks on the critics of psychoanalysis, Freud's statement of 1925 appears very moderate.

John Steiner, a Kleinian psychoanalyst, characterizes three types of bad reasons for criticizing psychoanalysis: genuine lack of understanding of the nature of psychoanalysis, rivalry among competitors for scarce resources, and envy. Of the latter he writes:

> The third type of attack is more difficult to deal with because it is motivated by envy. The aim here is to discredit and hence destroy psychoanalytic psychotherapy, and the methods used are unscrupulous and scurrilous. The attacks often arise in individuals who have themselves had a longing to be understood, and many have either been in analysis or toyed with it before focusing their hatred on it. Others have become consciously or unconsciously aware of the shortcomings of their own work. This discrepancy between the kind of understanding which these critics can offer and that demanded by their patients is often difficult to bear. To be then confronted by psychoanalysts who believe they have a way of understanding the communications of their patients is extremely provocative. Envy induces hatred and often a perverse righteousness in a crusade to expose the falseness of analysis. [Steiner, 1985]

Freud at least was trying to understand his critics in the context of the history of ideas—their opposition to psychoanalysis was part of a general reaction against the biological mysticism that dominated German medicine in the early part of the nineteenth century and that had been swept aside by Darwin and Pasteur. Freud's insistence on the scientific status of psychoanalysis was essential if it was to be distinguished from vitalism, mesmerism, and other quasi-mystical systems. Steiner's speculation on the psychological mechanisms of the critics of psychoanalysis is much more dangerous, not least because his criticisms can be so easily turned against him and, by association, against psychoanalysis itself. Perhaps psychoanalysis is envy-provoking, and psychoanalysts no less prone to self-righteousness than are its critics; and it is characteristic of closed systems of thought that they disqualify their critics rather than take their arguments seriously.

The context of thought, whether historical or psychological, is, however, an important element in trying to understand it, and one that is of special interest to psychoanalysts. Why is opposition to, and defence of, psychoanalysis so violent? This is itself a phenomenon needing explanation. One possible explanation is that underlying the controversy over psychoanalysis and psychotherapy in general are crucial differences of value, which genuinely do pose threats to the protagonists.

When psychoanalysis started, it challenged many of the prevailing beliefs about sexual morality. The recognition that there may be a connection between neurosis and the repression of sexual impulses, and that the undoing of repression may lead to health, was deeply disturbing. But, as the Scottish philosopher David Hume wrote:

> There is no method of reasoning more common, and yet none more blameable, than in philosophical debates to endeavour to refute any hypothesis by a pretext of its dangerous consequences to religion and morality. When any opinion leads us into absurdity, 'tis certainly false; but 'tis not certain an opinion is false, because 'tis of dangerous consequence. [Hume, 1739]

When psychoanalysis started, it was widely regarded as morally and politically subversive, as well as having a revolutionary novelty. This led to the widespread condemnation and vilification of its practitioners, which in turn produced an equally strong, almost religious, fervour on the part of its supporters. To a certain extent, we are still experiencing the legacy of these events. Furthermore, psychoanalysis has not altogether lost its subversiveness.

Perhaps the key issue today is not sex, but science. The controversy over psychoanalysis is part of a wider debate over the nature of scientific enquiry itself. Psychotherapy poses a challenge to scientism—in particular, to a narrowly defined "scientific" medicine and psychiatry that ignores questions of motivation and emotion. Just as the early psychoanalysts wished to explore sexuality while retaining a strong sense of morality, so today psychoanalysis sees the mind as a legitimate arena for rational non-mystical enquiry, while remaining true to the values of science taken in its broadest sense.

One result of this is that it is extremely difficult to form a balanced, objective view of the scientific status of psychoanalysis and psychotherapy. Not only is the material necessarily somewhat elusive, but it is important to be constantly aware of the dangers of being guided by non–truth-centred motives.

We have not attempted to consider the full weight of philosophical debate about the scientific status of psychotherapy. Our main conclusions from this brief account are that three characteristics of psychotherapeutic theory which have been seen as inherent weaknesses—the elusiveness of its potentially falsifiable hypotheses, the wide use of explanations in the alternative, and the tendency to question critics' motives for their beliefs—are hard to avoid in any enterprise that attempts to offer such a comprehensive explanation of and cure for human psychological misery. But is psychotherapy effective? This, for most people, is the decisive issue, rather than whether psychotherapy is strictly speaking a science, a pseudo-science, or perhaps an art.

Does psychotherapy work?

One of the most persistent worries expressed by critics of psychotherapy is the possibility that any good results it may achieve are a result not of the truth of psychotherapeutic theory or the aptness of its technique, but of the personal influence that the therapist has over the patient. This problem is not unique to psychotherapy. Modern medicine relies almost exclusively for evaluation of the efficacy of drugs on the *double-blind controlled trial*, in which an active treatment is compared with an inert but similar therapy, with both patient and prescriber remaining ignorant, until the trial is over, of which is which.

Michael Balint, a psychoanalyst who pioneered the use of psychotherapy in general practice, compared psychotherapy with drug therapy: "The doctor is a drug; the question is in what dose he should be prescribed, and with what frequency, and for which conditions" (Balint, 1957). If the doctor or therapist *were* a drug, evaluation of the effectiveness of psychotherapy would be relatively straightforward. Double-blind controlled trials could be mounted, and the results of active treatment compared with those of an inert placebo. If those given psychotherapy failed to show significantly more benefit than those who did not receive it, then serious doubts would be cast on psychotherapy's claim to be an effective treatment. But psychotherapy is not like that, and therein lies the rub for would-be psychotherapy researchers.

A psychotherapist is not a drug

It is worth considering the ways in which the therapist is *not* a drug. First, unlike drugs, therapists and the therapies they deliver do not work in one linear direction. Rather, therapy consists of a number of different tacks, one of which more or less predominates. Tape recordings of therapeutic sessions reveal that what therapists actually do often differs significantly from what attempts to formalize their practices would suggest that they do. Some analytic therapists, for example, can be found giving advice to their patients, whilst cognitive therapists, whose primary allegiance is behaviourism, not infrequently encourage expression of feelings or make interpretations of unconscious motivation.

Second, each therapist, even if she comes out of the same training "bottle" as others, is in an important sense unique. One therapist cannot be directly substituted for another in the way that a pill can. Modern medicine matches pill to *disease*, whereas psychotherapy depends on the establishment of a relationship between *people*, which may take precedence over both the technique of the therapist and the ailment of the patient.

This leads to a third difference, and the one that has aroused the greatest controversy among the researchers studying psychotherapeutic effectiveness. In pharmacotherapy there is an essential distinction between the *psychological* aspect of *believing* that a drug will help (the placebo effect), which in about 30 per cent of subjects will produce a perceptible alleviation of symptoms, and a *pharmacological* effect attributable to the physiological action of the drug. In psychotherapy, placebo and active principle, although still theoretically distinct, are not readily separable. An active drug can be surreptitiously slipped into someone's tea and still, unlike a placebo, have a pharmacological effect. A double-blind trial offers the patient either tea or sympathy and so tries to tease out which is the more essential ingredient. But in psychotherapy, the "tea and sympathy" are inextricably linked because the interest, attention, and compassion of the tea ceremony are inseparable from psychotherapy itself. A "correct" interpretation, given in a hostile way, will be ineffective. An unpalatable drug, if swallowed, will be no less effective than a sugared pill.

Unlike drug therapy, psychotherapy consists of a combination of general or *"non-specific"* features such as interest, compassion, and reliability, together with *particular* techniques like interpretations in psychoanalysis, or behavioural directives in behaviour therapy. Charles Rycroft (1985) is critical of the tendency among psychoanalysts to overvalue the importance of interpretations in producing change, in contrast with the "re-moralizing effect" (Frank, 1973) of these non-specific elements in therapy:

> Every correct interpretation, even when it is, as it should be, entirely free of reassurance or suggestion, contains within it a whole number of additional implicit communications about the analyst and his attitude towards the patient. In addition to enlightening the patient about, say, his phantasies or defences, it also indicates that the analyst is still present and awake, that he has been listening and has understood what the patient has been talking about, that he remembers what the patient has said during the present and previous sessions—and that he has been sufficiently interested to listen and remember and understand. [Rycroft, 1985]

A final distinction between a therapist and a drug is central to the above discussion, and indeed to the whole of this book. Drugs are chemical substances aimed at the physiology of those who ingest them. Therapists and their patients are *rational agents*. The outcome of therapy depends on a number of psychological factors distinctive of *people*—motivation for change, conscious and unconscious psychological forces—for which there is no pharmacological equivalent.

We may conclude, therefore, that a strict double-blind trial of psychotherapy, analogous to a drug trial, is probably impossible. This does not mean, however, that attempts to evaluate psychotherapy should be abandoned.

Good and bad psychotherapy research

A practical illustration of the possibilities and limitations of psychotherapy research is provided by a study of marital therapy by Michael Crowe designed to compare the effects of different therapies (Crowe, 1978). The researcher himself treated thirty-six couples, twelve of whom received analytic marital therapy, twelve behaviour therapy, and twelve "placebo" therapy, which consisted of "chats" with no specific content. He was a respected researcher, committed to behaviour therapy, holding no particular brief for analytic work. The results were unsurprising. Each type of therapy had some good outcomes; behaviour therapy did best and "placebo" worst, while analytic therapy was intermediate.

This study can be criticized on two grounds. First, double-blind conditions are impossible to achieve, since the therapist's expectations inevitably interfere with the therapeutic process. Second, it has been shown, unsurprisingly, that therapists do best when working in a therapeutic mode with which they are familiar and sympathetic (Luborsky et al., 1986). Crowe's study may reveal as much about the researcher as it does about different forms of marital therapy.

On the other hand, the Crowe study is a genuine attempt to tease out some of the subtleties intrinsic to psychotherapy research. It represents part of the growing attempt to overcome some of the obstacles to valid testing which we have discussed.

In another study, the Sheffield-based British researchers David Shapiro and Jenny Firth found that both behavioural and analytic therapy were highly effective in reducing neurotic symptoms over an eight-session period of treatment, and that this improvement was sustained at three-months follow-up (Shapiro & Firth, 1987). The therapists in this study were working according to "behavioural" and "analytical" guidelines, to increase the chances that the therapy was really practised according to the designated methods. Both types of therapy achieved good results: the behaviour therapy worked rather faster, whereas the analytic therapy resulted in fewer relapses.

We have cited these studies in order to contrast the subtlety and detail of their findings with the cavalier generalizations that have often been bandied about by partisan psychotherapy researchers of one persuasion or another.

The outstanding example of this is that scourge of dynamic therapies, Hans Eysenck. Although he appears not to have personally carried out any research on psychotherapy, he has been, for over thirty-five years, one of the leading exponents of the view that dynamic psychotherapy does not work. His original article on the subject in 1952 compared the published results of psychoanalytic psychotherapy with spontaneous remission rates for neurotic disorders (Eysenck, 1952). It claimed that, given the tendency of neurosis to improve with time irrespective of treatment, and given the prolonged nature of psychoanalytic therapy, any improvements claimed by psychoanalysts were invalid, since they could have taken place spontaneously. Thus he concluded that the therapy must be ineffective. This sweeping conclusion has subsequently been conclusively refuted, the spontaneous improvement rate in neurosis being in fact about half that which results from psychotherapy (Lambert, Shapiro, & Bergin, 1986). But Eysenck was not even entitled (tentatively) to draw the conclusion from the evidence available to him at the time— for his research findings rested on three crucial errors.

First, his choice of evidence was highly selective: he ignored those studies that suggested that neurotic symptoms can be very persistent, and often do *not* resolve spontaneously without therapy.

Second, he failed to distinguish between psychoanalysis proper, which often lasts for several years, and psychoanalytic psychotherapy which, although usually much briefer, lasting for as little as ten weeks, can lead to significant symptom reduction sustained over time.

Third, he misrepresented the *aims* of psychotherapy, which are not, as he suggests, solely concerned with the relief of presenting symptoms. This relief usually starts to occur fairly early on in therapy. But, as we stressed in chapter one, psychotherapy has more ambitious goals: it aims to help the patient become more autonomous and to achieve more satisfying relationships, to enhance self-esteem, and to prevent further breakdown. These take longer to achieve and, had Eysenck looked at them, which he did not, significant differences between untreated groups and those receiving therapy might well have emerged.

It is interesting that more recent research has forced those who wish to dismiss psychotherapy to shift their ground. Since 1952 numerous studies have demonstrated that psychotherapy is effective, both in removing symptoms and in achieving some long-term goals, and produces much more improvement than results from spontaneous remission (Lambert et al., 1986). The anti-psychotherapy argument has now shifted from the original claim that there is no difference between therapy and no treatment at all, to the claim that specific psychotherapy is no better than placebo therapy. According to Eysenck:

> Even now, thirty years after the article in which I pointed out the lack of evidence for therapeutic effectiveness, and some five hundred extensive investigations later, the conclusion must still be that there is no substantial evidence that psychoanalysis or psychotherapy have any positive effect on the course of neurotic

disorders, *over and above what is contributed by meaningless placebo treatment.* [Eysenck, 1983; italics added]

We have already discussed some of the difficulties inherent in applying the placebo concept to psychotherapy and have suggested that, given the nature of psychotherapy, it is hard for placebo therapy ever to be "meaningless". Readers of this authoritative statement by Eysenck might be surprised to learn that the *authors* of the study from which he derived his conclusions, Smith, Glass, and Miller, summarize their evidence as indicating the "consistent, positive and large effects of verbal psychotherapy compared to placebo treatment" (Smith, Glass, & Miller, 1980). Their study, which was based on averaging the results of a large number of controlled outcome studies, by a procedure known as "meta-analysis", concluded that the average "effect size" of psychotherapy was around 1 standard deviation unit. *This means that the average psychotherapy patient did better than 85 per cent of control subjects. Put another way, 70 per cent of psychotherapy patients improved, while 30 per cent did not; 30 per cent of control subjects improved "spontaneously", while 70 per cent did not* (Karasu, 1986). "Control subjects" here mean patients who are offered brief nonspecific "chats" or unfocused discussion groups, some of which may have some unavoidable psychotherapeutic content that would, if anything, bias the results against psychotherapy.

To conclude from these and similar studies that analytic therapy is ineffective suggests that Eysenck and his more recent co-attackers such as Shepherd (1979), Wilkinson (1986), and Webster (1996) have already decided that psychotherapy is no good and are simply scratching around for any snippet of information that will apparently support their case.

Psychotherapy research is difficult. Eysenck's approach is simply to sweep aside the difficulties and draw the conclusions he is looking for. Some supporters of psychotherapy have reacted to this by stating the view that psychotherapy is in principle unresearchable. Their view is that psychotherapy research is so difficult, and so likely to lead to trivial conclusions far removed from the profundities of therapy, that it cannot be worthwhile, and even that it should not be attempted. They claim to be dealing with imponderables, not suitable for scientific enquiry, and have seized on the crassness of Eysenck's criticism to dismiss the whole enterprise as irrelevant to their purposes. Consider, for example, this defensive posture adopted by John Steiner:

We need to explain that we cannot promise specific therapeutic results, but we can properly offer psychotherapy as the treatment of choice to the patients we accept. We have to acknowledge that the results of psychoanalysis and psychotherapy cannot be demonstrated by the type of trials which are helpful in testing drugs, because these are unsuitable for the testing of treatments which involve human characteristics and concerns. To attempt trials of this kind we must strip our observations of the very meaning which we believe makes them of value. Sometimes, as an analogy, I suggest that similar problems would arise if we wanted to prove that the late works of Dickens were superior to his early ones. I have no doubt that this is true and that every lover of Dickens would agree, but attempts to prove it scientifically, say by computer counts of mean sentence length, would render the exercise meaningless. [Steiner, 1985]

Although we would agree that drug trials and tests of psychotherapy are very different, we would not accept Steiner's argument that it is impossible to test "treatments which involve human characteristics". For Steiner adopts the narrow scientistic view of research which we reject. Let us consider an important example: George Brown and Tyrill Harris have shown, using subtle interviewing and statistical techniques, that central factors in determining whether a woman becomes depressed in the face of loss or life difficulties are her early childhood experience and the quality of her marital relationship (Brown & Harris, 1978). This finding is consistent with psychoanalytic theories of depression and can properly be used as part of an argument for marital therapy in the treatment and prevention of depression (see chapter four). There is no reason to suppose that psychotherapy cannot be properly researched, or that the search for objective evaluation is bound to be misguided.

It is difficult for a lay person to form a rational judgement about the effectiveness of psychotherapy, because alleged experts have such radically conflicting positions. Because psychotherapy is concerned not just with technique, but with *values* that arouse strong passions and that may conflict, there is a tendency for protagonists on both sides to vilify their opponents, to be selective in their research, and to resort to hyperbole. We believe that there is sufficient sound research to show that psychotherapy can be effective in a number of ways and circumstances. We do not aim to convince those implacably opposed to psychotherapy, but we do hope the uncommitted will be more ready to accept the conclusions that we summarize below.

What psychotherapy can and cannot do

Psychotherapy is effective. There are now several well-designed studies that have repeatedly shown that patients with anxiety or depressive symptoms, or mild to moderate personality difficulties, improve significantly compared with controls, when treated with psychotherapy (ably summarized in Roth & Fonagy, 1996). We have referred to Shapiro's Sheffield project (Shapiro & Firth, 1987) and would also point to Weissman's well-known depression project (Weissman, Sholomokas, & John, 1981). The latter showed that depressed women treated with sixteen sessions of interpersonal therapy (concentrating on current problems) improved markedly, especially in their "social functioning", that is, in their relationships with their immediate family, ability to form friendships, join clubs, and so on, compared with non-treated controls.

This study illustrates the importance of specifying what is meant by "outcome". A narrow focus on symptom removal disqualifies an important part of what psychotherapy aims to achieve. An individual might emerge from analysis with symptoms controlled rather than eliminated, but feeling and being more autonomous, realizing her own limitations, and understanding some of the causes of her problems. This would be a positive outcome, even though the symptoms were not entirely eliminated. Symptom check-lists are an easy but crude research tool, compared with the questionnaires and semi-structured interviews needed to measure the improvements in relationships, self-esteem, and maturity that psychotherapy aims for.

The widened and strengthened social relationships that come about as a result of psychotherapy may also have a preventive effect against future breakdown. Prevention is especially hard to research, but there is good evidence that family therapy can reduce the chances of relapse in schizophrenia (Leff, Kuipers, & Berkowitz, 1982), and that both interpersonal therapy (IPT) and cognitive behavioural therapy (CBT) can delay relapse in depression (Roth & Fonagy, 1996). Psychotherapy as a form of preventive care is an active if complex area of psychotherapy research.

Psychotherapy is not ALWAYS effective and can do harm. Deterioration in psychotherapy is well-documented (Mays & Frank, 1985). This has been used tendentiously in arguments both for and against psychotherapy. Supporters argue that it must be a powerful treatment if it can make people worse as well as better; opponents, that it is dangerous and best avoided.

Most medical treatments, both effective and ineffective, can, if improperly used, be harmful. Deterioration in psychotherapy is usually the result of either poor selection of patients or bad therapeutic practice. Not all patients are appropriate subjects for psychotherapy, or for a particular type of therapy. Intensive analytic therapy with patients suffering from schizophrenia can, for example, precipitate rather than prevent psychotic breakdown. It takes the very special pleading of an analytic enthusiast to argue that *this is* desirable. Equally, patients firmly entrenched in a sick role of multiple neurotic or psychosomatic symptoms may resist psychotherapeutic attempts to pull them towards autonomy. There are also those who might appear to need psychotherapy but are unlikely, without modifications of psychotherapeutic technique, to benefit, due to lack of motivation, severity of illness, or educational deprivation (see chapter four).

The qualities in a therapist most likely to cause deterioration are a cold, aloof, and detached attitude on the one hand, or seductive behaviour on the other. As we discuss in chapter six, the effective therapist is objective but not cold, warm but not seductive. The need to protect vulnerable patients from inappropriate therapies and bad therapists will be fully explored in the second half of this book.

Psychotherapy and drug therapy are not mutually exclusive. It is commonly thought that drug treatment makes people inaccessible to psychotherapy by dampening down the very feelings that are the raw material of therapy. This is not so. It has been shown, for example, that in depression a combination of anti-depressants and psychotherapy produces a better outcome for social functioning and symptom removal than either alone (Klerman, 1986). One of the aims of psychotherapy is to promote emotional autonomy, and the need to use drugs can indicate a lack of autonomy. However, there may be occasions where a good outcome in psychotherapy might include an acknowledgement by the patient that she *does* need, for example, anti-psychotic drugs, just as a diabetic is made more, rather than less, autonomous by acknowledging a need for insulin.

There is no one major type of psychotherapy that is consistently more effective than others. Luborsky's "Dodo-bird verdict" (from *Alice in*

Wonderland)—*"everyone* has won and all shall have prizes"—has yet to be refuted (Luborsky, Singer, & Luborsky, 1975). Research has generally failed to demonstrate the superiority of any major type of therapy over others. Freudian psychoanalysis is not superior to Jungian analysis, although it may well suit some individuals better; in one study, patients randomly assigned to group marital or individual psychotherapy did equally well compared with controls (Pilkonis et al., 1984); in a major study, behaviour therapy produced comparable results overall to those achieved by a form of dynamic therapy (Sloane et al., 1975). This surprising, and perhaps unpalatable, finding for those therapists who are wedded to their own particular model has to be considered together with the next point.

Therapists, as opposed to therapies, differ significantly in their effectiveness. Some therapists consistently produce better results than other therapists (Luborsky et al., 1975). This applies whatever school the therapist belongs to. Effectiveness is also only poorly correlated with length of training—training probably producing less variation in effectiveness than personal qualities. The view of Carl Rogers that accurate empathy, non-possessive warmth, and honesty are the essential attributes of an effective therapist has stood the test of time (Rogers, 1957).

There is also evidence that technique is important as well as the personal qualities of the therapist. A study by Luborsky which looked in detail at what therapists said in sessions showed that there was a correlation between good outcome and therapists who stick consistently to a particular model of therapy (Luborsky et al., 1975). David Malan, in his study of brief analytic therapy, found a correlation between good outcome and the therapist's ability to adhere consistently to the analytic model, and so make transference interpretations, although this finding has been challenged (Malan, 1963). In general, the evidence seems to suggest that the combination of adherence with flexibility is the best recipe for effective therapy (Roth & Fonagy, 1996).

The Equivalence Paradox. Stiles, Shapiro, and Elliott have dubbed the above two apparently contradictory findings "The Equivalence Paradox" (Stiles, Shapiro, & Elliott, 1986): most therapists believe strongly in their model, and do best if they stick to it and hone it, yet outcome is not crucially dependent upon which model it is. We shall offer three explanations for this apparent paradox.

First, there is the issue of "non-specific factors" in therapy. All effective therapies, whatever their orientation, contain elements that include implicit hope, an attempt to understand and make sense of psychological stress, and respect and concern for the patient as a human being. If these were predominant in determining outcome, then one would expect the personal qualities of the therapist to be important, but it would not matter which model she followed.

A second explanation might be that, psychologically speaking, all roads lead to Rome. This follows from the way in which mental states are organized hierarchically with reciprocal feedback between levels. To oversimplify: behaviour is linked with specific plans and strategies, which in turn connect with deeper patterns of feelings and attitudes. Change at one level has inevitable effects at another. Masters and Johnson's behavioural sex therapy, for example, directs partners to spend more time stroking one another. This in turn is likely to lead to increasing trust and improved emotional communication, and this may ultimately influence deeper levels at which basic attitudes towards relationships between the sexes may begin to change. Conversely, analytic therapy will start at the "basic attitude" end of the hierarchy and hope that this will ultimately be reflected in enhanced sexual communication. Behaviour therapy may have more immediate impact, and so work faster, but possibly with less reverberative and so less lasting effects. Cognitive therapy occupies an intermediate position, tackling "basic assumptions" as well as encouraging patients to change their behaviours. Analytic therapy may have less immediate impact, but greater resonance. Each kind of therapy is appropriate to its own circumstances; neither is definitely superior.

A third possible explanation of the Equivalence Paradox is that it is a research artefact. Outcome studies necessarily give standard treatments to groups of diagnostically different cases, which one might expect, on average, to give similar results irrespective of treatment modality. In clinical practice, following an assessment interview, therapists try to find the best match between patient and problem, available therapies and therapists. In group therapy, for instance, more extrovert individuals do better with behavioural methods while introverted types fare best with analytic approaches.

This is relevant to the question of *eclecticism* in psychotherapy. Eclecticism is good when it applies to patients, less so when practised by therapists. A range of therapies is needed to suit different psychotherapeutic problems; model-hopping therapists who offer their patients a hodgepodge of treatments will get less good results than those who stick to one familiar method.

The Equivalence Paradox certainly does *not* show that specific psychotherapies are ineffective, or that the differences between therapies are unimportant.

Outcome studies in psychotherapy come up against an inherent methodological problem because, although *physiologically* similar, and thus comparable in a drug trial, human beings are *psychologically* different in many of the ways that matter for psychotherapy. This problem is not insuperable because we do all share certain vital interests: in the avoidance of pain, for example, and, as we argue in chapter three, in autonomy, self-esteem, and satisfying relationships. Furthermore, methods can be found to measure success in achieving these more personal objectives. But both subtlety and good will are required if these methodological difficulties are to be overcome.

Is psychotherapy cost-effective?

In the two major sections of this chapter, we have discussed the case against psychotherapy in terms of abstract-seeming questions as to whether psychotherapy can claim to be scientific and whether it can be shown to be effective. As far as the *practical* issues of this book are concerned, however, the key debate has, as the anti-psychotherapy psychiatrist Michael Shepherd put it,

> ... to do more with economics and medical politics than with the niceties of scientific inquiry. . . . [In the United States] psychotherapy is big business, and its exponents are mainly in private practice where their income depends largely on third party payments from medical insurance. . . . This state of affairs has already resulted in widespread lobbying for the inclusion of mental disorder in insurance policies and in extensive advertising through the mass media. In addition, because the practice of psychotherapy remains without firm professional credentials, understandable but unseemly competition has developed be-

tween rival mental health professionals—psychiatrists, psychologists, social workers, nurses and counsellors of various persuasion. And, since the recent move towards making federal funds for psychotherapy dependent on proof of efficacy and safety, the suggestion that a psychotherapist is little more than a placebologist [sic] must be, in Maher's pithy phrase, as welcome as a tax auditor at a business lunch. [Shepherd, 1979]

Resources for all types of social care are scarce, and governments are increasingly wary of "throwing money" at social problems. Under these circumstances the question of whether psychotherapy is cost-effective assumes great importance. If psychotherapy were obviously far more expensive than other treatments, that would, so far as the case for expanding psychotherapy is concerned, be almost as bad as discovering that it did not work at all. Practitioners and policymakers alike have an ethical responsibility to ascertain whether particular kinds of treatment are cost-effective.

At present the level of publicly funded formal psychotherapy services is very low, although calculating the full extent of psychotherapy is difficult, given the diversity of definitions (NHSE, 1996). We calculate that within the British National Health Service (NHS), for example, funding of formal psychotherapy amounts to perhaps £10 million within a total health service budget of £17 billion (i.e. 0.068 per cent!). This compares with the overall allocation to psychiatry of around £2 billion.

The economic case against psychotherapy would be that it should be accorded a low priority in public expenditure because it offers poor value for money. In its most extreme form, the criticism is that since psychotherapy is ineffective anyway, it is quite wrong to spend public money on it. The private sector may flourish, since it would be wrong to restrict the liberty of individual citizens, but state funds should not be wasted on useless treatments. A less extreme version of this argument is that although psychotherapy can be effective, the time and effort that it requires do not justify spending public money on "an undefined technique applied to unspecified cases with unpredictable results" (Shepherd, 1979).

We have already argued that psychotherapy *can* be shown to be effective, so the extreme version of the argument does not require further discussion. As regards the less extreme version, there are few cost–benefit analyses of psychotherapy. Evidence is to be found, however, that suggests that psychotherapy *can* be cost-effective, even within the comparatively narrow parameters of hard-nosed health economics. If patients effectively treated with psychotherapy show a reduction in their use of medical and welfare resources, then the money spent may have been better employed than appears at first sight. An important study from the Cassel Hospital in Richmond, London, which offers in-patient psychotherapy for severe cases of neurosis and personality disorder, suggests just this (Rosser et al., 1987). A health economist calculated the total cost to the Exchequer of patients before and after therapy. Many of the patients were unemployed before treatment and had received considerable amounts of largely ineffective treatment and support from multiple medical and social agencies. Where the outcome of psychotherapy was successful, patients reduced or stopped altogether their involvement with helping agencies, and many obtained jobs. The saving in public expense produced by a good outcome far exceeded the total cost of treatment. The net gain for the entire sample of twenty-eight patients, of whom two-thirds were judged to have improved, was about £500,000. More recently, a similar study was conducted at the Henderson Hospital, which specializes in treating people with personality disorders, often those who, as a consequence of their personality, have run into difficulties with the law (Dolan & Norton, 1996). The Henderson is run as a therapeutic community, based around group analytic therapy. Residents stay for several months, up to one year. Here, too, patients who stayed for more than three months did well. This type of therapy is not cheap (about £40,000 for a year's treatment), but within two years of discharge these people had *saved* the Exchequer more than had been spent on them by entering the treatment programme.

An interesting aspect of the Henderson study is that it was undertaken at a time when the Health Authority was seriously considering closing the unit altogether. The Government was so impressed that they are now actively encouraging the establishment of similar units across the country. The use of this type of calculation is familiar in other branches of medicine and justifies, for example, the cost of expensive procedures such as open-heart surgery and kidney transplants, although it is perhaps worth noting that coronary artery surgery for angina, a generally accepted and practised form of treatment, has not been shown on *trials* to produce better results than the much cheaper medical treatments with pills (Brooks, 1988).

Units like the Cassel provide the psychotherapeutic equivalent to major surgery. There is also now increasing evidence for the cost-effectiveness of using psychotherapeutic techniques in general practice, where the psychotherapy can reduce or avert the need for hospital admission, reduce subsequent rates of consultation with doctors, and lead to a decrease in the consumption of psychotropic drugs (McGrath & Lowson, 1986).

These studies indicate that psychotherapy is cost-effective and not just for those with "minor" disorders that would be likely to improve without treatment. Our society contains large numbers of the "walking wounded": patients with depression, anxiety states, suicidal behaviour, chronically disturbed relationships, and psychosomatic conditions. There is good evidence that many of these could be effectively and cost-effectively helped by psychotherapy, were it available. Unlike some defenders of psychotherapy, we believe that health economics has a significant contribution to make to the development of psychotherapy services.

We take issue with psychotherapists who see a cost–benefit approach as intrinsically antipathetic to the spirit of psychotherapy, and who reject it on the grounds that the subtle and delicate issues of the human spirit cannot be reduced to balance sheets. While they are right to maintain that these issues cannot be *reduced* to balance sheets, policymakers cannot avoid making trade-offs between desirable objectives. Hitherto, psychiatry has lost out in competition for resources with those specialities where there are more powerful vested interests, both medical and commercial, notably the drug and medical supply industries, who are not shy to use cost–benefit analysis to support their claims. A similar process has happened in miniature within psychiatry. Psychotherapy is the "soft" end of psychiatry and, as such, is vulnerable to resource starvation, just as psychiatry loses out through being the "soft" end of medicine.

Conclusion

Psychotherapy is effective and is what many patients want, expect, and need when they experience emotional distress or illness. It is not necessarily expensive. Yet it is currently available only to the few. Investment in psychotherapy, based on sound economic arguments, is necessary if this need is to be met.

Having accepted this, however, it is important to realize that cost–benefit analysis for psychotherapy is, like the other areas of psychotherapy research, especially difficult and complex. One factor that makes this so is that psychotherapy aims not just at symptom removal, but at more fundamental personal changes, whose value is itself the subject of controversy. If it *could* be shown that psychotherapy was a cheaper and more effective form of symptom removal than alternative treatments such as tranquillizers and antidepressants, the case for more extensive psychotherapy would be relatively straightforward. We have cited research that suggests that, in some important areas, it is.

However, it is not on such a claim that our main arguments for expanding psychotherapy are based. The main function of this chapter has been to counter the dismissive generalizations of the more extreme opponents of psychotherapy. We have argued that the scientific status of psychotherapeutic theory is no worse than that of any *psychological* explanation of the life of human beings; that psychotherapy *does* work—both in the removal of presenting symptoms and in promoting growth in autonomy and self-esteem and improving personal relationships; and that psychotherapy can be cost-effective and is not obviously more expensive than other treatments, even as far as symptom alleviation is concerned.

We can now proceed to discussion of the most important reason for seeking to expand psychotherapy, which is independent of psychotherapy's claims to be a cheap or effective method for alleviating symptoms. As Anthony Ryle puts it:

> The central aim and value of psychotherapy . . . is that of enlarging people's ability to live their lives by choice. While the removal of symptoms is a worthwhile act, and is sometimes all the patient requests, the nature of psychologically derived symptoms is such that wider aims are nearly always implied. These aims are achieved by enabling patients to acquire a more accurate and fuller experience in place of muted, denied, or distorted experience, and by reducing those aspects of life that are lived by compulsion or evasion, and extending those that are lived by desire and intention. [Ryle, 1982]

Psychotherapy does not aim at the *suppression* of symptoms. While it may aim at symptom *removal*, it also has wider goals, including the promotion of emotional autonomy, which, in turn, leads to greater self-esteem and more effective personal relationships. Are these further benefits something that should be regarded simply as a luxury for those able and willing to pay for them, or are they benefits that citizens of a civilized society should be able to expect? This is the subject of the next chapter.

CHAPTER THREE

Is psychotherapy
a luxury?

As we saw in the preceding chapter, one source of opposition to psychotherapy comes from those who hold it to be at best an unscientific form of treatment, and at worst simply an excuse for unscrupulous charlatans to exploit the misery or gullibility of their customers. We argued—against these and more measured criticisms—that psychotherapy is effective and, from the standpoint of scientific credibility, fares no worse than other kinds of psychological enquiry or psychiatric treatment.

We ended by looking briefly at whether psychotherapy is cost-effective. The studies we cited show that it can stand up well, even on its weakest ground—the areas of symptom alleviation and severe mental disorder. However, studies of cost-effectiveness require some assumptions of value—about the relative importance of potential

The main argument in this chapter was worked out in R. Lindley, "Psychotherapy as Essential Care", in G. Fairbairn & S. Fairbairn (Eds.), *Psychology, Ethics and Change* (London: Routledge & Kegan Paul, 1988). The authors would like to thank the editors and publishers for permission to use material which appeared first in that work.

goals. Once there is agreement about goals, the task is then to discover the most efficient method of achieving them. We believe that the strongest reason for seeking to expand psychotherapy is that it offers its beneficiaries something of vital importance which cannot be provided by other treatments or social interventions.

There is a worry shared by opponents, and even some supporters, of psychotherapy, that the problems it seeks to alleviate are too ephemeral to be regarded as the proper province of public funding. In short, psychotherapy is, from this view, just a luxury.

Should psychotherapy be regarded, like personal swimming pools and world cruises, as basically a luxury, available to those who want to indulge themselves in it, and have the ability to pay for it; or should it be treated as a basic form of care to which everyone, at least in the relatively affluent "developed" nations, should be entitled?

Should psychotherapy be publicly funded?

The public funding of an activity, in a democracy, requires justification since ultimately it is paid for by coercive taxation of the citizenry. In order for psychotherapy to be the sort of activity that should be subsidized by the taxpayer, it would have to be a treatment that offered its beneficiaries something of *substantial* importance. Otherwise, it would be wrong for publicly funded health authorities to invest their scarce resources in psychotherapy, for the demand for health care resources always greatly exceeds supply. This view is strongly expressed by Dr M. Hunt, a correspondent to the *British Journal of Psychiatry*:

> The present controversy about psychotherapy seems to me a great deal of talk about new methods of treating sprain whilst ignoring the fractures. As long as there is [sic] insufficient manpower and resources to deal adequately with the diseased and the disabled, it would seem that the distressed and dissatisfied warrant a lower priority, rather than the reverse. . . . I would . . . suggest that, when the last psychotic patient is reasonably free of distressing and troublesome symptomatology, has reasonable personal hygiene and appearance, and has adequate diet, occupation and living conditions, then psychiatrists can concentrate on psychotherapy to the exclusion of all else, since there will be nothing else left to do. [Hunt, 1985]

This argument purports to appeal to an assumption that we, and probably most of our readers, would accept. It may be expressed in many ways, but the one we prefer is this: *justice requires equal consideration to be given to the interests of all those affected by public actions and policies.* Let us call this the *Principle of Equal Respect*.

If, following a serious road accident, it were possible for surgeons to save either the life of one victim or the hand of another, but not both, other things being equal it would be right to save the life, wrong to save the hand—irrespective of the wealth, social class, ethnic origin, or gender of the victims. The reason most of us find this so obvious is that we accept the Principle of Equal Respect. Not to save the life would be indicative of a failure to treat the person whose life was lost with the respect that should be shown for the interests of everyone, regardless of status.

Adherents of political views from across the political spectrum appeal to the Principle of Equal Respect. There is obviously *political* advantage to be gained from such appeals, since, by purporting to give consideration to the interests of all, politicians are more likely to solicit the support of all. This, however, gives no reason for a deliberating agent to *believe* in the Principle. The rationale of the Principle is rooted in moral views—for example, the Kantian principle according to which all people should be treated as "ends in themselves" rather than simply as means to the ends of others (Kant, 1795), or the conviction that the interests of no one *individual* are intrinsically more valuable than those of any other (Bentham, 1789).

We shall, at various stages in our argument, appeal to the Principle of Equal Respect. We shall not, however, offer a general defence of the Principle, for three reasons: (1) it would be a lengthy digression in a book on psychotherapy; (2) where we appeal to the Principle, it is to weaker versions of it, to which we assume most of our readers will assent; and (3) the Principle is well defended elsewhere (Baker, 1987).

Hunt's argument makes implicit use of a weak version of the Principle which would command widespread support. Few would want to question the view that, other things being equal, it is right, at least within the domain of public responsibilities, to give priority to more serious needs, wrong to ignore them in order to attend to more trivial needs. For a society to ignore the more serious needs of one group in order to provide trivial benefits for another is indicative of an unjust failure to treat the former with a proper respect. The satisfaction of anyone's more basic interests is, in itself, of more moral importance than the satisfaction of anyone's less basic interests.

It is also true that, as a rule, the treatment needs of the psychotic, the mentally "diseased" and "disabled", are more basic than those of the (merely) "distressed" and "dissatisfied" who might typically seek psychotherapy.

However, the Principle of Equal Respect, even when combined with a recognition that the needs of the psychotic for help are typically greater than those of the (merely) "distressed" and "dissatisfied", does not rationally compel policymakers to conclude that psychotherapy should be abandoned, suspended, or curtailed until all psychotics have been cured.

To establish such a conclusion, it would be necessary to show not only that the less fundamental needs of one group should be left until the more basic needs of every other group have been met, and that it is impossible adequately to fund both psychotherapy and the (non-psychotherapeutic) treatment of the more seriously mentally ill, but also that devoting more resources to psychotherapy would actually be detrimental to the more seriously ill. We hope to show that these claims, when analysed, are highly dubious. Let us consider them in turn.

Scarce resources and a decent minimum

Hunt's argument raises a general issue that directly leads on to questions of justice. The important moral question seems to be: "Should we, as a matter of principle, concentrate our scarce mental health resources exclusively on the most serious needs of the psychotic, to the exclusion of the less pressing needs of the 'merely distressed'?" Hunt assumes that the answer is "No". Suppose that there were four people each asking for a share of a loaf of bread that you had to distribute. If two were actually starving, whereas the other two were just a bit hungry, other things being equal you should divide the loaf between the starving, giving nothing to the others.

What is phoney and dangerous about the use of such arguments in the field of public care is that it presupposes that there is a loaf of fixed size, to be fought over by all possible beneficiaries. Of course, there are limits on the resources that a society at a given level of affluence and technological development *can* direct to the care of the needy. But unless, in a given society, that limit is being approached, it is hypocritical for the controllers of public finances to claim that psychotherapy can be funded only if care for the most seriously ill is jeopardized. The allocation and distribution of resources for meeting people's needs tends to be determined by political bargaining, often producing a result that is, from a moral point of view, arbitrary. The hypocrisy of the above trade-off argument is that its appeal to moral principle ("give greater weight to more pressing needs") masks the fact that decisions about how much of the gross national product will be allocated to caring for the needy are often taken on political rather than moral grounds. It is accepted (on moral grounds) that provision should be made for saving the lives of those with kidney failure by renal transplant *and* for improving the lives of those with arthritis by hip replacement; similarly, there should be adequate treatment both for psychotics *and* for those suffering from neurosis.

The shortcomings of the trade-off argument may be seen in the field of housing, where it would be perverse to argue that government-funded home-improvement grants for the poor should be withdrawn until homelessness has been abolished. It is true that the needs of bathroom-less house-dwellers are less urgent than those of the homeless, but to look at housing problems in this way is to divert attention from the fact that both the homeless and the bathroom-less have serious needs which could and should be met in a society as affluent as the United Kingdom or the United States without placing an undue burden on public expenditure overall.

Given a society where there is sufficient wealth for large numbers of people to live at a standard that is *far* above what is recognized as a decent minimum, it should not be necessary to accept the perverse Robin Hoodist principle, implicit in this reasoning, of taking away from the poor to save the destitute.

The main moral case for seeking an expansion and widening of availability of psychotherapy is that psychotherapy offers patients benefits that are at least as important as other benefits that are non-controversially regarded as the responsibility of society to provide. One of the main reasons for supposing that society has a responsibility to ensure that its citizens have adequate health care is that such care is a prerequisite for attaining a decent minimum quality of life. This decent minimum will vary from society to society, according to overall affluence and level of technological development. Modern Western societies *are* sufficiently affluent and developed to be able to make psychotherapy available to all who need it, as well as attending properly to more urgent needs. A crucial reason for seeking the expansion of psychotherapy is that *psychotherapy* may be, for many people, a prerequisite for a decent minimum quality of life.

But even if it were *not* possible properly to fund both psychotherapy and non-psychotherapeutic treatments of the more seriously mentally ill, it is not clear that the Principle of Equal Respect *would* require that psychotherapy be sacrificed in order to fund these other treatments.

Does more psychotherapy mean worse treatment for the seriously disturbed?

An implicit assumption made by Hunt and other critics is that devoting resources to psychotherapy is against the interests of the more seriously ill, and that a decision to reduce investment in psychotherapy would actually benefit the psychotic, whose needs, all agree, are most pressing. Consider this view of psychoanalysis put forward by one of its more implacable opponents, whom we discussed in the previous chapter:

> Psychoanalysis is highly expensive and limited in its application to integrated, wealthy and functioning individuals, who are interested in learning more about themselves, or who need to relate their personal problems to a strong figure. The disconcerting aspect of psychoanalysis is that it drains resources from the care of seriously mentally ill patients. [Wilkinson, 1986]

This is rather a caricature of psychoanalysis, which in any case is but one form of psychotherapy, and the most expensive at that. Anyway, our case for more publicly funded psychotherapy does not rely on the claim that *psychoanalysis* should be regarded as part of essential care for everyone. However, the assumption that more psychotherapy means worse treatment for the seriously mentally ill does not survive even modest scrutiny.

It is by no means clear that in the long run the seriously mentally ill need suffer from an expansion of publicly funded psychotherapy: indeed, they could benefit from it. There are at least three reasons for this.

First, psychotherapy, by helping its patients to develop self-esteem and emotional autonomy, indirectly yields substantial benefits for society as a whole. In simple economic terms, distress and dissatisfaction are very costly. When people are chronically unhappy with themselves and their lives, they are unlikely to contribute effectively to society, either through their work or their family. At one extreme, the distress of a top administrator of an organization could lead to poor decisions being taken, or lower morale to the great detriment of the organization as a whole. On the other hand, effective psychotherapy might enable a "problem" person or family to become more self-reliant and less of a drain on scarce welfare resources. In both cases, therefore, it could plausibly be argued that there would be a net economic gain to society, and so funding psychotherapy could, if policymakers chose to make it, be an indirect *investment* for better treatment for the mentally ill. If the merely dissatisfied and distressed are denied treatment, that will exacerbate their dissatisfaction and distress and they will lose; but so too might people who are worse off than they.

Second, there is some, admittedly as yet limited, evidence that psychotherapy has a preventive role. If timely psychotherapy could prevent patients in the early stages of an illness from becoming more severely ill, then it would not be wrong to make psychotherapy available, since this would release extra resources for care of the severely ill by reducing their numbers.

Finally, even if, for some reason, it was thought that the less seriously mentally disturbed should be left to cope until the more seriously disturbed patients had been cured, this should not necessarily hit psychotherapy in particular. Although psychotherapy is neither the only nor perhaps the main treatment that can help the severely disturbed, there is evidence that it can benefit them. Luborsky and his co-workers have shown that the chances of drug addicts giving up heroin are greater for those treated with a combination of psychotherapy and detoxification, than for patients given detoxification alone (Luborsky et al., 1985). Leff and his team found that only 15 per cent of schizophrenics treated with family therapy relapsed in the year following admission, compared with the 60 per cent who relapsed without therapy (Leff & Vaughn, 1984); and other studies have shown that *none* of a group of schizophrenics given psychotherapy and drugs relapsed, compared with 40 per cent of those on drugs alone (Tarrier, 1988). Certain severe personality disorders respond positively only to psychotherapy, and in some depressed patients psychotherapy can prevent relapse and even suicide.

We have already mentioned the findings of the Cassel project in the previous chapter, in which it was shown that the psychotherapeutic treatment of severe cases of neurosis and personality disorder saved the Exchequer a large amount of money (Rosser et al., 1987).

Inadequate funding for psychotherapy harms those with the greatest needs by denying them effective treatment, as well as doing indirect harm in the long run by placing an extra burden on the Exchequer.

Needs and flourishing

If psychotherapy should be available to people in the way that basic medical care and education are available, then psychotherapy must offer a way of satisfying *some* basic needs. But what does this mean? A need is a necessary condition for something else. Thus to say that *x* needs *y* is to say that *x* cannot attain something else that is good for it without *y*.

In the most general terms, a "basic need" is a necessary condition for something or someone to be a good specimen of its kind. Thus the needs of a living thing are determined by what it is for that kind of living thing to flourish or "do well". Obstacles to flourishing or well-being (we shall use the terms interchangeably) can either be *internal*, in which case we speak of the organism being diseased, or external (environmental). The two are not as easily separable as one might think, for unfavourable environmental conditions can generate and sustain disease, and diseased individuals can effect their environment in a negative feedback loop. This makes the boundaries of caring professions such as medicine difficult to define. The doctor's prime concern is to combat disease. But to do so it may be necessary to intervene in her patient's environmental circumstances.

Although all living things, including people, have a variety of basic needs, these are not all of the same importance. Less important needs become a priority for an organism's flourishing only when the more important needs have been satisfied. The needs of sentient creatures—that is, beings which are capable of experience—are especially complex, since as well as any purely biological needs for survival and successful reproduction they have needs specifically associated with their capacity to be the subject of experiences. Sentient creatures have all kinds of good and bad experiences. By virtue of their capacity for experience, we may properly speak of sentient creatures having interests (Singer, 1979). They have interests in having good experiences and avoiding bad, whether or not these are co-extensive with purely biological needs. For a sentient creature to flourish requires, at least, that its life be not full of pain and, to a certain extent, be pleasant.

Human beings, with obvious exceptions such as young infants and the severely brain-damaged, are more than merely sentient in that they possess *self*-consciousness and the ability to choose what to do, even if these abilities are constrained. Following a long philosophical tradition, we may therefore characterize human beings, apart from the exceptions referred to above, as *rational* creatures— meaning not that they lack emotions, nor that they always act for the best possible reasons, but merely that they have the capacity to act for reasons, whether these are good or bad. In other words, human beings are capable of choice. Only creatures that are rational in this sense can be *irrational.*

Because human beings have the capacity to choose, their interests have an extra dimension of complexity over those of creatures that are merely sentient. Like them, we have biological needs and an interest in pleasant experiences. In addition, there is the possibility of *distinct* interests arising out of our capacity to *choose.* It is difficult to produce a plausible *general* theory of human interests, because there may be conflicts between these different levels of interest. Just as pleasant experiences may conflict with biological needs, so what we would choose may conflict with what would produce the most pleasant or least painful experiences.

Certainly since the time of Socrates controversy has abounded over what it is for human beings to flourish. It has proved impossible to settle the matter by argument from self-evident premises and agreed facts alone; and it is unlikely that a genuine proof for a particular view will ever be found. The question "What is it for a human being to flourish?" might *look* like a scientific or technical question, and indeed there are certain scientifically determinable physiological conditions that are necessary for a human being to do well as an organism. But we are here concerned with what is essentially an ethical question.

Although this is an ethical question and may admit of no technical or universally compelling answer, it must not be dodged, for all social policy rests on *some* assumption about what constitutes a good (enough) life for a human being, and this makes at least implicit appeal to a conception of human flourishing. Moreover, it is possible to make rational comparisons between rival conceptions without appeal to supposedly absolute moral truths. Our method for attempting this is to bring into the open the less obvious, and frequently ignored, consequences of accepting one or another conception. Such a method, like any attempt at rational persuasion, appeals ultimately to assumptions that themselves are not questioned. In order for such a strategy to succeed, it is enough if the two parties share some common value, and the successful party can show that only on his conception can that value be properly realized or promoted.

Human well-being

Autonomy: personal and emotional

As we mentioned in chapter one, there are many kinds of psychotherapy, and the range of techniques employed by different therapists is vast. Nevertheless, there is a common theme in the overwhelming majority of therapies: namely, a recognition of the intrinsic value of *personal autonomy*. Joel Kovel, offering advice to would-be psychotherapy patients as to which form of therapy to choose, writes: "the one value that can be emphasized in the selection and conduct of a therapy is the pursuit of free, autonomous choice. Neurosis enslaves . . ." (Kovel, 1978).

What is autonomy? Autonomy literally means "self-rule", and has its origins in the ancient Greek city-states, where granting a dependent state *autonomia* meant allowing it a degree of devolved self-government. The term has been transposed to apply to individual people as well as collectivities. Autonomy, in the context of psychotherapy, implies taking control of one's own life. The deep-seated desire for autonomy is captured in this statement by Isaiah Berlin:

> I wish my life and decisions to depend on myself, not on external forces of whatever kind. I wish to be the instrument of my own, not of other men's acts of will. I wish to be a subject, not an object; to be moved by reasons, by conscious purposes, which are my own, not by causes which affect me, as it were, from outside. I wish to be somebody, not nobody, a doer—deciding, not being decided for, self-directed and not acted on by external nature or

by other men as if I were a thing, or an animal, or a slave incapable of playing a human role, that is, of conceiving goals and policies of my own and realising them. . . . I wish, above all, to be conscious of myself as a thinking, active being, bearing responsibility for my choices and able to explain them by reference to my own ideas and purposes. [Berlin, 1969]

In this statement, Berlin, who is writing as a political philosopher, posits a distinction between an "internal" self or agent striving for autonomy and "external" forces that may control or thwart this wish. The importance of his account for psychotherapy (and perhaps of psychotherapy for his account) is that many people, especially those seeking psychotherapy, are frustrated not by their circumstances but by themselves. The "external nature" by which they feel controlled comprises their own impulses and feelings; the "causes" that affect them are internal, although they may be experienced as alien and unwanted. Psychotherapy enhances autonomy because it brings these internal "external" forces within the orbit of the acting, thinking, and (we would add) feeling, responsible self. This idea is contained in Freud's imperative definition of the aim of psychoanalysis as "where id is, there ego shall be" (Freud, 1923b), or in Bettelheim's re-translation, "where *it* is there *I* shall be" (Bettelheim, 1983). We shall call this state "emotional autonomy".

As we mentioned in chapter one, emotional autonomy does not mean isolation or avoidance of dependency. On the contrary, the lonely schizoid individual who preserves his "independence" at all costs may well be in a state of emotional heteronomy, unable to bear closeness with another person because of inner dread and confusion. A similar state of emotional heteronomy affects the psychopath, who is unaware of the feelings of others. The emotionally autonomous individual does not suppress her feelings, including the need for dependence, but takes cognisance of them, ruling rather than being ruled by them. In Freud's important qualification of his principle, he likens the ego to a horseman and the id to the mount, and points out that at times, in order to control one's horse, it has to be given its head.

It would in any case be an idle wish to want to be *completely* free from outside forces of whatever kind, not least because we are finite creatures whose powers and freedoms are limited by each other and by natural limitations. However, many obstacles to self-determination can, in principle, be overcome without detriment to other people.

Of particular relevance to this book are *internal* barriers to self-determination. It is not unrealistic to seek to become someone who takes more responsibility for her choices, and is able to explain them by reference to her own ideas and purposes.

Autonomy is a matter of degree, and heteronomy—that is, lack of autonomy—may be more or less serious. Nobody can be completely autonomous, but, for a variety of reasons, many people are far less autonomous than they need be.

From the cognitive point of view, one common cause and manifestation of heteronomy is simple ignorance. A person whose important decisions are based on mistaken beliefs is not in control of her life. A clear example of this would be a young child who, on the promise of sweets, is persuaded to get into the car of a complete stranger, unaware of the dangers. The main remedies for ignorance are education and experience. But psychologically troubled individuals are not just ignorant (although ignorance may be part of their trouble); they are also emotionally disturbed.

Emotional disturbance produces irrationality, and irrationality is a form of heteronomy. There are two distinct kinds of irrationality, although they may be difficult to disentangle in practice, since one kind rarely occurs without the other. The first is *theoretical* irrationality, where a person's beliefs are not suitably proportional to the evidence available to her. The second is *practical* irrationality, where, in spite of having rational beliefs about the relevant features of her situation, a person deliberately chooses to do something that, given her own beliefs and goals, is self-defeating or counter-productive.

Psychotherapy helps its patients by promoting their emotional autonomy. It does so by putting them in touch with their emotions and by reducing theoretical and practical irrationality. It produces a "man that is not passion's slave"; not someone who is emotion-less, but rather someone who is no longer enslaved by emotion-generated heteronomy. This is, in part, a developmental process, providing an opportunity for emotional growth towards maturity to occur; in part, an educational process, coming to understand what emotional forces are at work within one; and, in part, a moralizing process, effectively giving one the strength to do what one really judges to be best.

Being autonomous clearly has a certain instrumental value. For heteronomy is an obstacle to successful pursuit of one's projects. It deprives a person of the pleasures that success would bring, and it produces its own pain. But autonomy is sometimes painful, and ignorance is said to be bliss: the responsibility that accompanies the recognition that one's actions really are a true expression of what one values can be awesome.

If the distinctive contribution of psychotherapy is that it helps to promote emotional autonomy, which is a constitutive element of overall autonomy, then the value of psychotherapy is likely to depend on the value of autonomy. Is autonomy an essential part of human well-being?

We consider here two rival nineteenth-century views of human nature and argue that the importance of psychotherapy's goals is derivable from acceptance of the more plausible of the two. According to the first, the only intrinsic goods for people are pleasant experiences and the absence of painful ones. This view, associated with Jeremy Bentham [1748–1832], formed the cornerstone of classical utilitarianism and was particularly influential during the early nineteenth century. The other view, most closely associated with Bentham's pupil John Stuart Mill [1806–73], whilst acknowledging the unique value of pleasure, distinguishes between qualities of pleasure and includes autonomy as an essential part of human well-being. We shall compare the views, starting with Bentham's, in particular looking at what implications the different conceptions might have for social policy. An appreciation of the relative shallowness of Bentham's conception helps to reveal the importance of the goals of psychotherapy.

Bentham

Human beings are sentient, so to have pleasant and pain-free experiences is at least partially constitutive of human well-being; but are there not any other constituents? There are certainly many things other than pleasure and the absence of pain which are thought to be good—a decent roof over one's head, good health, security, variety—the list is endless. But, according to the Benthamite, their worth consists only in the fact that they contribute to people's pleasure. We shall in the rest of this chapter, where the context permits, use "pleasure" as a shorthand for "pleasure and the absence of pain". Bentham believed that pleasure is the *only* non-derivative good for human beings, and that for a person to flourish is simply to have a life filled with the greatest possible amount of pleasure.

According to the Benthamite view, the aim of society in general, and of the caring professions in particular, should be to maximize pleasure. Pleasure and pain are regarded as psychological states which are comparable and measurable according to their duration and intensity. This view is consistent with the Principle of Equal Respect to the extent that no person's (or indeed sentient creature's) pleasure is in itself more significant than anyone else's. Nobody is to count for more than anyone else.

Bentham's ethical hedonism was certainly influential in helping to free Victorian society from superstitious adherence to principles of conduct that had long since outlived their usefulness. It provided a common standard against which any government policy, indeed any proposed conduct whatsoever, could be evaluated.

However, Bentham's conception of well-being and its accompanying morality, by treating all pleasures and pains as strictly commensurable, ignores the structural complexities of being a person. It cannot capture the dignity of personhood, and it allows the possibility of sacrificing some people's welfare totally, in order to promote the more peripheral interests of a large number of others. In principle this could be taken to justify gladiatorial contests, provided that the crowds, who enjoyed such spectacles, were large enough.

On this view the only way of improving someone's well-being is to increase her pleasure, and the only way of harming someone is to decrease it. The Benthamite version of the utilitarian "Greatest Happiness Principle" is an injunction to maximize pleasure. It does not *in itself* matter how the pleasure is distributed, although in practice Benthamite utilitarianism does have a limited egalitarian tendency since, with a few notable exceptions, the worse off someone is the greater increase in pleasure she will receive from a given size of material benefit. There is, however, no limit to a person's pleasure, and no matter how well-off someone is, a further gain in *pleasure* is no more nor less significant than a gain of similar magnitude for someone far worse off. Benthamite utilitarianism contains no *essentially* distributive principles of justice.

It is important for a defender of psychotherapy to be able to reject the Benthamite view of human well-being.

If pleasure and the avoidance of pain were the only constituents of human well-being there would be little reason to give anything but the lowest priority, so far as public responsibility goes, to a supposed service that makes little contribution to the promotion of pleasure or the reduction of pain. Although it is clear that psychotherapy can make a contribution to a reduction of pain and an increase in pleasure, pleasure as such is not its ultimate justifying aim, and in many cases the success of psychotherapy for someone is not measured in increases in Benthamite pleasures. Freud, for example, in a famous statement about his early work, characterized his main objective with hysterical patients not as the elimination of pain or the production of pleasure, but rather as the transformation of "hysterical misery into common unhappiness" (Freud, 1895d). Freud's aim was the overcoming of hysterical heteronomy (denial and repression) by greater awareness and the re-experiencing of childhood traumas in the safety of the therapeutic relationship. He did *not* aim directly to help hysterics to adjust, or to get them to "feel better".

It might be claimed that for Freud autonomy was only of instrumental value, because Freudian psychotherapy as a treatment for hysteria can be an instrument, among others, for increasing pleasure. In this respect, psychotherapy would be no different in kind from, and might be more expensive than, say, an "anti-hysteria" drug (antidepressants can sometimes help with hysteria).

Such a claim would be misguided for at least two reasons. First, hysteria is not necessarily "painful". Freud's recognition of the primary and secondary "gains" from hysteria acknowledge this—the primary gain being the avoidance of anxiety, the secondary gain the sympathy and interest aroused in others by the "sufferer". Second, Freud appeared to value autonomy as a category quite separate from, and sometimes in conflict with, pleasure. For Freud, autonomy has intrinsic value.

Freud's belief that "common"—that is, "non-hysterical"—unhappiness is in itself preferable to hysterical misery conflicts strongly with the Benthamite view. For Bentham, becoming free of neurotic patterns of behaviour is, like everything else apart from pleasure, of merely instrumental value. From the point of view of an individual's well-being, the only thing wrong with irrationality and heteronomy is that they may tend to make one's life less pleasant.

If nothing other than pleasure had intrinsic value, the case for a publicly funded expanded psychotherapy service would be greatly weakened: there already exists a wide range of drugs that are in many cases more efficient and effective at *pain relief* and *euphoria production* than is psychotherapy. Nevertheless, even if Bentham's views were accepted, psychotherapy could still have an important though comparatively small role to play. As we have seen, psychotherapy can be cost-effective, especially when combined with other treatments, for relieving the pain of severe mental disorder; it may have a preventive role; and in a number of cases brief psychotherapy can be a cheaper treatment for effectively reducing psychological pain than is drug therapy.

Our view—that psychotherapy should be regarded as an *important* part of essential care—does, however, require a rejection of the Benthamite conception of human flourishing. Although it is not possible to *prove* that the Benthamite conception is wrong, we think that it has consequences that, on reflection, should render it unacceptable to nearly everyone, including those inclined to reject the case for psychotherapy. To see this more clearly, let us consider what a world of Benthamite human flourishing might be like.

Perhaps a close approximation to the ideal Benthamite society, where the net balance of pleasure over pain is about as great as could be expected, is described in Aldous Huxley's dystopian novel *Brave New World*. A policy of well-planned positive eugenics, combined with comprehensive behaviour modification and subliminal learning programmes throughout childhood, ensures that almost the entire population is well suited to whatever role is regarded by the rulers as socially desirable for it to fill. There is material abundance; wars are obsolete; personal antagonisms are at a minimum; and people are able to enjoy, through developments in advanced technology, a wide range of thrilling experiences. Anxiety, anger, depression, and other painful or anti-social psychological states are kept firmly under control through the free use of *soma*, a powerful psychotropic drug that replaces unpleasant thoughts and feelings with an overwhelming euphoria, often accompanied with harmless fantasies. Even the pains of growing old are abolished:

> Now such is progress—the old men work, the old men copulate, the old men have no time, no leisure from pleasure, not a moment to sit down and think—or, if ever by some unlucky chance such a crevice should yawn in the solid substance of their distractions, there is always *soma*, delicious *soma*, half a gramme for a half-holiday, a gramme for a week-end, two grammes for a trip to the gorgeous East, three for a dark eternity on the moon; returning whence they find themselves on the other side of the crevice, safe on the solid ground of daily labour and distraction,

scampering from feely to feely, from girl to pneumatic girl, from
Electro-magnetic Golf Course to . . . [Huxley, 1955]

On any plausible calculation, Huxley's Brave New World is an
exceedingly pleasurable place. It is certainly far more so than any
known society on Earth. Yet is it a society that we should seek to
emulate? One powerful reason for not trying is that there are countless pitfalls that could make any such plans go disastrously wrong.
We have not yet developed an effective *soma* which is free of harmful
side-effects, and there are, anyway, legitimate fears about the
accountability and responsibility of the power-holders in such a
highly organized society.

But the most powerful argument against moving towards a Brave
New World is surely that, even if it were possible, it would be a
nightmarish world rather than an ideal society. Indeed, Huxley
stated in the Foreword to the 1950 edition of his novel that he had
written it as a warning of the horror that might befall the Western
world if urgent steps were not taken to resist it.

The fact that the inhabitants of Brave New World enjoy pleasant
lives cannot on its own explain the repugnance of that society for
those who, like most people, believe that pleasure is an intrinsic
good. If that society is really repugnant, therefore, it must be because
there is something so seriously wrong with it as to outweigh the
enormous advantages of such high levels of pleasure.

What *is* wrong with it? Essentially it is this. The quality of the
inhabitants' lives is seriously impoverished due to lack of autonomy.
Rather like Milton's Adam and Eve before eating from the Tree of
Knowledge, the citizens of Huxley's Brave New World are childishly
naïve, their emotional lives lack depth, and their personal relationships are superficial. Their pleasure is largely based on illusion; they
are, by design, highly conventional. Although they are not driven by
unruly emotions to act irrationally, they have extremely low levels of
cognitive autonomy (they are heteronomous in respect of their beliefs). There is hardly any scope for the development and expression
of individuality.

The fact that people are rational creatures, capable of acting in
pursuit of goals set by their own conceptions of a worthwhile life,
gives them interests that the merely sentient lack. The widespread
abhorrence felt for Huxley's society suggests that there is more to a
flourishing human life than simply having a succession of pleasant

experiences. Perhaps foremost among our other vital interests is an interest in making good use of our rational capacity, in developing and exercising our autonomy.

A general complaint against authoritarian, highly centralized political regimes is that they deny their citizens autonomy. Even if under a system of total control people *would* live more pleasant lives, and make fewer mistakes than free citizens, they would not be thought to be more flourishing human beings.

So we reject the Benthamite conception of human well-being, and now consider the rival view of John Stuart Mill.

Mill

According to Mill, the development of personal autonomy is necessary for human well-being. There are two ways in which this could be so. It might be that without autonomy it is impossible to attain the other constituents of a good life; on the other hand, autonomy could be thought to be *intrinsically* desirable.

Autonomy has instrumental value because being autonomous and exercising autonomous choice is a necessary *means* for attaining pleasure. However, although there is *some* positive correlation between degree of autonomy and level of pleasure, the correlation is not perfect, as *Brave New World* illustrates. Indeed, it is possible that increasing someone's autonomy could also increase her pain, particularly pain associated with anxiety.

Another way in which autonomy is a necessary *means* to other things that are intrinsically good is that deep personal relationships and various other goals may be frustrated by lack of autonomy. Someone who has failed to resolve his dependency on his parents may find it difficult to develop and sustain a mature loving relationship with another adult. This lack is not necessarily painful, as Paul Simon's lyrics suggest: "I am a rock, I am an island. And a rock feels no pain. And an island never cries." On the other hand, putting things right, which might mean making the person more aware of the true forces that motivate her, could increase her pain, particularly in the short run. However, it may be better to have loved and felt pain than not to have loved at all; and without autonomy this kind of mature loving may be impossible.

The Millian view of human well-being recognizes the instrumental value of autonomy. But it goes further, holding that autonomy is itself *partially constitutive of well-being*. In other words, a life lacking in autonomy is in itself impoverished, irrespective of the pleasure and pain it may hold.

Of course, it is not possible to *prove* that autonomy is one of the constituents of human flourishing. However, its importance has been stressed by moral and political theorists at least since the Enlightenment. The belief that human flourishing includes autonomy is certainly not the invention of psychotherapists in search of customers. Let us now examine in more detail the Millian conception, which has a crucial role in the case for psychotherapy.

Mill's Choice Criterion of well-being

Mill remained a utilitarian throughout his life, believing in the "Greatest Happiness Principle". However, as we have said, he developed a conception of "happiness" or "well-being" which departed radically from Bentham's, and included autonomy amongst the constituents of true human happiness. Mill believed not only that autonomy is an intrinsic good, but that people who have a high degree of autonomy actually do better (are flourishing more) than those who, though somewhat deficient in autonomy, are well-endowed with Benthamite pleasure. He argued that those who have attained a high level of autonomy would prefer to retain it, even if to do so is, on balance, painful.

For Mill, the ultimate test of what constitutes human flourishing is appeal to people's preferences as expressed in the choices they make. Pleasant experiences are intrinsically good, since people choose them for their own sake, without any ulterior motive. However, there are other things besides pleasant experiences that people want for no ulterior reason. These, by the Choice Criterion, should also be regarded as intrinsic goods.

It is not, however, plausible to claim—and Mill did not claim—that the good for individuals is fixed *simply* by consulting their actual choices or preferences. For choices and preferences may be impaired. Someone who has lived a very sheltered and protected life might prefer to remain at home, cut off from the outside world. On Mill's view, this would not show that staying at home was the best thing for that person. What would be good for her is fixed by what she would choose, *were* she properly informed about the nature of the choice and the other options available.

Similarly, it cannot be inferred from her extreme reluctance to go out that it is in the best interests of an agoraphobic to stay indoors. Ignorance and irrationality can deny people the chance even to be aware of opportunities that, were they aware of them, they would very much want to pursue.

In a famous passage about the preference for an active, self-aware, autonomous life over an existence of mere contentment, Mill wrote:

> Whoever supposes that this preference takes place at a sacrifice of happiness . . . confounds the two very different ideas, of happiness, and content. It is indisputable that the being whose capacities of enjoyment are low, has the greatest chance of having them fully satisfied; and a highly endowed being will always feel that any happiness which he can look for, as the world is constituted, is imperfect. But he can learn to bear its imperfections, if they are at all bearable; and they will not make him envy the being who is indeed unconscious of the imperfections, but only because he feels not at all the good which those imperfections qualify. It is better to be Socrates dissatisfied than a fool satisfied. [Mill, 1861]

For Mill, our capacity for rational choice is perhaps the most morally important feature of human nature, being the *sine qua non* of freedom. We have the capacity to act in pursuit of our own self-chosen—or, if not self-chosen, at least self-scrutinized and endorsed—projects. We potentially have the capacity to use our rationality to resist immediate inclinations to believe or act. For Mill, the ultimate criterion of what constitutes human well-being is *whatever would be preferred by people whose choices were not constrained by ignorance and irrationality.* He believed that the overwhelming majority of people whose choices were not so constrained would not be prepared to abandon their autonomy, even for huge gains in pleasure.

On this view, then, in order to decide what it would be for people to flourish, we must address ourselves to what they would choose, if their choices were not constrained by heteronomy. The sorts of things that almost everyone would so choose, although the order of preference might vary, include: accomplishment, choosing one's own course through life, making something out of it according to one's own lights, being in touch with reality, enjoyment, and deep personal relationships. For a full discussion of this subject, see Griffin (1986).

Happiness and the Principle of Equal Respect

Another crucial difference between Millian and Benthamite treatments of human happiness is this: Bentham's view, as we have seen, treats pleasures and pains as strictly commensurable—distinguishable ultimately only by quantitative measures of intensity and duration. Thus, for Bentham, "the greatest happiness" is a state of the world where there is as much pleasure as possible. One criticism of this view is that individual *people* seem to drop out of the moral calculus. Mill never explicitly rejected this formula, and at certain places in his writing seems to have endorsed it. However, there is also evidence of a quite different view of happiness—especially in his essay *Utilitarianism*. Here Mill defines happiness as:

> . . . not a life of rapture; but moments of such, in an existence of few and transitory pains, many and various pleasures, with a decided predominance of the active over the passive, and having as the foundation of the whole not to expect more from life than it is capable of bestowing. A life thus composed, to those who have been fortunate enough to obtain it, has always appeared worthy of the name of happiness. And such an existence is even now the lot of many, during some considerable portion of their lives. The present wretched education, and wretched social arrangements, are the only real hindrance to its being attainable by almost all. [Mill, 1861]

For Mill, society's goal should not, apparently, be simply to produce the greatest balance of pleasures over pains, or even the greatest number of pleasant autonomous experiences. As well as speaking of the greatest happiness, Mill frequently wrote about "the general happiness" as being the chief goal at which society should aim. On the basis of this analysis, which is admittedly only one strand in Mill's thought, "the general happiness" is a goal that could be attained were society only organized properly. This differs from the Benthamite conception, according to which there is in effect no such state as "being happy", and according to which any one increase in pleasure is as important as any other equally large increase, no matter how relatively well-off the beneficiaries were at the outset. The Millian conception—at least as expressed in the above quotation—has a built-in respect for the individual and a recognition of a fairly strong version of the Principle of Equal Respect. "The general happiness" is a state in which happiness is "general", that is, a state in which as many people as possible have attained the state described above. There is a level of well-being that is such that, beyond it, further gains in welfare are morally insignificant compared with the moral importance of attaining it. The chief responsibility of a society should be to ensure that everyone, or at least as large a proportion of the population as possible, has reached this state.

To summarize: on the Millian view of human well-being, pleasurable experience is but one of the constituents of human well-being. This follows from the Choice Criterion together with plausible empirical assumptions about what people would choose were their choices unconstrained by irrationality and ignorance. One of the most important of these other constituents of human well-being is autonomy itself. Being autonomous means having one's choices unconstrained in the above way, and thus being in a position to understand what is good for oneself. Furthermore, a relatively high level of autonomy is a prerequisite for other intrinsic goods, notably deep personal relationships. The citizens of Huxley's Brave New World lack the understanding of themselves or others to enable them to form anything more than shallow, insignificant relationships with each other. Although pleasure and a relatively pain-free existence are part of human well-being, it is often worth sacrificing some pleasure to increase autonomy. Finally, there is an attainable level of well-being, called "happiness" by Mill, which society ought to help as many people as possible to attain.

As we said earlier, we do not pretend to offer a *proof* of the special intrinsic value of autonomy, and are certainly aware that Mill's claim that autonomy is part of human well-being is not self-evident. The claim relies on the Choice Criterion, but the privileged position accorded to autonomy by Mill is already implicit in the Choice Criterion itself, and cannot therefore be established simply by application of that criterion.

Perhaps it is a mistake to try to provide an ultimate foundation for a conception of human well-being. Much of our subsequent argument about psychotherapy relies on the claim that autonomy is an essential constituent of human well-being. It is legitimate and not futile to rely on this assertion provided that the claim is plausible, and in, fact accepted by a wide section of those whom we are trying to convince about the value of psychotherapy. The above discussion has been intended to establish this plausibility, and to show that the view is in fact widely accepted.

We would further hope to persuade the doubtful that the conception of human well-being as requiring autonomy is reasonable, by pointing out that it is presupposed by commonly accepted moral arguments in defence of liberal democracy. It is only because autonomy is so important that benevolent dictatorships and Brave New World *are* so abhorrent. If opponents of psychotherapy can realize and appreciate the significance of accepting that autonomy is part of human well-being, significant progress will have been made.

Autonomy, essential care, and psychotherapy

Extreme individualists, such as Robert Nozick (1974) might claim that everyone should look after themselves and that there is no reason why the better-off in a society should be constrained to help the worse-off. To argue against this extreme position would take us beyond the scope of this book. We are starting from the liberal democratic consensus view, according to which a civilized society should, so far as possible, guarantee a basic minimum quality of life or decent human existence for its members.

There is no a priori method for computing, for any given society, exactly where that level should be. It is fairly uncontroversial, however, that the top priority should be given to the prerequisites, where attainable, of a decent human existence. It is on these grounds that we believe that everyone should have basic food, shelter, and clothing. In addition, health care should be available to all, on the grounds that good, or at least reasonable, health is a requirement for a decent human existence (see Daniels, 1985).

Many of the "essentials" for a decent human existence are in fact means for staying alive and avoiding pain. Within the field of medicine, for example, it is recognized that society has a responsibility to ensure that there is adequate funding to support research into and treatment of cancer. On the other hand, although saunas and jacuzzis are pleasant, and may even improve health, they are properly not regarded as matters of public responsibility. Rather, they are luxuries; for what they offer is not necessary for human flourishing.

According to the Millian view, which we endorse, autonomy is an essential part of human well-being. If this is so, then activities that are specifically directed towards the development, restoration, or maintenance of a reasonable level of autonomy should be regarded as important in the same way as many forms of basic physical health care. Many people, owing to adverse life experiences and failures to resolve deep-seated emotional conflicts, are unable to attain or sustain a reasonable level of emotional autonomy. For these people, psychotherapy offers the best and in many cases the only remedy.

According to a popular image, psychotherapy appears to be more the sort of activity that one would associate with an exclusive health-and-fitness club than a part of essential care. There are several reasons for this, which we discuss in more detail in the next chapter. One of the most important is that psychotherapy is very unevenly distributed, being readily available to, and sought by, only the socially and financially better-off. This, however, may reflect the widespread deprivation among the less well-off rather than providing just another example of luxuries being primarily available for the rich.

Psychotherapy and education: an analogy

Throughout the book we draw on analogies with education. Before the great education reforms of the nineteenth century, formal education was regarded as inessential for all but a privileged elite. However, the fact that in those days the majority of the population survived without education, and did not seek it, did not prove that education *was* just a luxury that should be available only to those whose parents could afford it. Similarly, although the "distressed and dissatisfied" can survive without psychotherapy, it may well be that they are being denied something that is at least of comparable value to standard medical care and basic education.

It is, of course, a big step from this to conclude that psychotherapy should be available to all those who need it, in the way that basic health services are at least supposed to be. Apart from questions concerning psychotherapy's efficacy, there is the intractable problem of the level of well-being that a society should aim to provide for as many of its members as possible. We cannot provide a general answer to such a question here. However, this is, according to our argument, no more of a problem for defenders of psychotherapy than it is for those who claim that education, housing, or health services should be available even for those unable to afford them. Because autonomy, reciprocal relations of love and friendship, self-esteem, and accomplishment are all parts of a good human life, psychotherapy should at least be able to set up a major stall in the market for scarce public care resources.

The main aim of this chapter has been to defend psychotherapy against one specific charge: that it is a luxury service, which should therefore be largely distributed according to social status and ability to pay. If psychotherapy does offer something essential to a decent human existence, then, by the same argument that is used to justify education and health care for all who need it, should there not be psychotherapy provision for all who need it? In the next chapter, we that develop the argument that there should be, and we also examine reasons for, and possible answers to, the inequitable distribution of psychotherapy.

CHAPTER FOUR

The unjust distribution of psychotherapy

We argued in chapter three that psychotherapy addresses basic needs, and we suggested that its distribution should not be determined by the ability to pay for it. It is our belief that in this respect psychotherapy should be regarded, like basic health care and education, as something that should be equally available to people according to need. This follows from the Principle of Equal Respect.

This Principle is really about well-being or flourishing, and it states that people should not be disadvantaged on arbitrary grounds. Of course, natural differences, which from a moral point of view are arbitrary, mean that it is not possible for everyone to flourish equally. A person born with severe spina bifida may never be able to achieve a level of well-being that approaches that of the able-bodied. A child who dies of leukaemia will have less of a good life, no matter what we do to help, than someone who lives out a normal healthy life. The crucial point is that scarce essential services should not be distributed on an arbitrary basis. To distribute health care or education simply according to ability to pay is to do an injustice to those whose needs for the services are great, but whose financial resources are small.

Justice, health care, and psychotherapy

Justice is consistent with inequality to the extent that it is not necessarily unfair or arbitrary that one person should, in certain respects, be better off than another. There are certain services, however, which, on widely shared views of justice, ought to be available to all, irrespective of wealth or relative power in the market-place. Examples include education, the protection of the law, and health care, but not personal swimming pools, world cruises, or second homes. What is the basis for this difference?

In a well-known article, Bernard Williams claims that medical care should be distributed to people simply according to their needs:

> Leaving aside preventive medicine, the proper ground of distribution of medical care is ill health: this is a necessary truth. Now in very many societies, while ill health may work as a necessary condition of receiving treatment, it does not work as a sufficient condition, since such treatment costs money, and not all who are ill have the money; hence the possession of sufficient money becomes in fact an additional necessary condition of actually receiving treatment. . . . When we have the situation in which, for instance, wealth is a further necessary condition of the receipt of medical treatment, we can once more apply the notions of equality and inequality: not now in connection with the inequality between the well and the ill, but in connection with the inequality between the rich ill and the poor ill, since we have straightforwardly the situation of those whose needs are the same not receiving the same treatment, though the needs are the ground of the treatment. This is an irrational state of affairs. [Williams, 1973]

On this view, health care should be distributed according to user need rather than ability to pay because the internal goal of health care is treatment of the sick. Similarly, it could be argued that the internal goal of education is imparting knowledge, skill, and wisdom and that consequently the proper ground for the distribution of education facilities should be educational need. If this were accepted, it would not follow that everyone would receive exactly the same education, or the same medical treatment; rather, that differences in people's education and health care would be determined by their differing needs. Could we simply extend Williams's argument to apply to psychotherapy distribution according to need?

Unfortunately, Williams's argument cannot, as it stands, be relied upon, since it has consequences that even those who accept its conclusion would find unpalatable. The structure of the argument is as follows: wherever a service has an internal goal, as, for example, medicine has the internal goal of curing sickness, it should be distributed in such a way as best to achieve that internal goal. Robert Nozick revealed the shortcomings of Williams's argument by asking a number of embarrassing questions:

> But why must the internal goal of the activity take precedence over, for example, the person's particular purpose in performing the activity? ... If someone becomes a barber because he likes talking to a variety of different people, is it unjust of him to allocate his services to those he most likes to talk to? Or if he works as a barber in order to earn money to pay tuition at school, may he cut the hair of only those who pay or tip well? Why may not a barber use exactly the same criteria in allocating his services as someone else whose activities have no internal goal involving others? Need a gardener allocate his services to those lawns which need him most? [Nozick, 1974]

What is special about education, medical treatment, and, as we have argued, psychotherapy is not that they are activities with internal goals, but rather that what they offer helps people to achieve a prerequisite for a decent human existence. The Principle of Equal Respect requires that more important interests should be satisfied before less important, irrespective of whose they are. Inability to avail oneself of gardening services does not threaten vital interests, unlike inability to secure medical attention. Nevertheless, not all medical services are equally important, and there may be certain peripheral treatments that should be regarded more like the gardening services. In arguing for medical care, education, or psychotherapy to be distributed according to need, it is implicit that there will be some cut-off points beyond which society's responsibility will rightly end.

Nozick is right to express concern for the freedom of practitioners as well as for the well-being of their beneficiaries. However, there need not be a serious conflict of interests between them in the areas with which we are concerned; there is no reason to suppose that the provision of basic psychotherapy services distributed according to user need would *seriously* invade the professional freedom of psychotherapists. For society to undertake a responsibility to provide health care or psychotherapy according to need does not have to impose any serious restrictions on practitioner freedom. Such an undertaking is not, for example, inconsistent with the preservation of a private sector of care. The most plausible objections to private care rely on appeals to the inadequacy of public provision. But adequate public provision is not, in itself inconsistent with private provision which might, perhaps, offer services that really *are* luxuries.

If basic psychotherapeutic care were provided according to user need, therapists who wished to remain Nozickian gardeners would be free to do so. But one could hardly expect society to invest in their services. On the other hand, those paid by public funds would have a social responsibility to provide a need-based service, and there would be no injustice to them in requiring that they provide a socially useful service.

We believe that psychotherapy, like medical care and education, should be available to those who need it, as part of the essential care for which society as a whole takes responsibility. As argued in the previous two chapters, psychotherapy offers its patients benefits that are, in their own way, as important for human well-being as those offered by education and much of what comprises standard medical practice.

There is, as we shall show, overwhelming evidence that psychotherapy is certainly *not* distributed according to need, and this should be a cause for great concern.

Class, mental health, and psychotherapy

When the *Titanic* sank in 1912, death was not evenly distributed (Hollingshead & Redlich, 1958). Among women on the first-class deck, only 4 out of 143 (3 per cent) were drowned; on the second-class deck 15 out of 93 women (16 per cent) died; while among the steerage passengers 81 out of 179 women (45 per cent) lost their lives. This class gradient in marine mortality neatly mirrored conditions that existed and continue to exist on shore. Some seventy years later, the Black Report, commissioned by the British Government, on *Inequalities in Health* showed

> ... marked differences in mortality rates between the occupational classes, for both sexes and at all ages. At birth and in the first month of life twice as many babies of "unskilled manual" parents (Class V) die as do babies of professional class parents

(Class 1) and in the next eleven months four times as many girls and five times as many boys. . . . A class gradient can be observed for most causes of death. [Townsend & Davidson, 1982]

The same applies to morbidity:

> Available data on chronic sickness tend to parallel those on mortality. Thus self-reported rates of long-standing illness . . . are twice as high among unskilled manual males and 2.5 times as high among their wives as among the professional classes. [Townsend & Davidson, 1982]

A similar gradient applies to psychiatric disorders, although this has been less thoroughly documented (Hollingshead & Redlich, 1958). Rates for most forms of mental disorder are greater among the working class—including schizophrenia, personality disorders, deliberate self-harm, substance abuse, and reactive depression.

The reasons for these class gradients in health are complex, and far from fully understood. Underlying these are two other gradients: adverse conditions of life, and the distribution and use of medical resources. On average, working-class people have a poorer diet, work harder, smoke and drink more, live in more stressful housing conditions, and are more exposed to environmental pollution than are middle-class people. In addition, recent work on stress as a factor in coronary artery disease shows higher morbidity and mortality in lower civil-service grades than in executive and administrative grades, even when diet, smoking, and other factors are allowed for (Lorion & Felner, 1986); this suggests that *lack of control* over one's life and working conditions, which is a form of heteronomy, is itself stressful and may be a contributory causative factor in disease. Unemployment, also concentrated in the lower social classes, is a further important class-related cause of ill health, both mental and physical: suicide and attempted suicide rates are considerably higher among the unemployed than among those in work.

While adverse living conditions produce greater morbidity among working-class people, the quality of medical care that they receive is generally inferior. Working-class women, for example, make far less use of preventive services such as ante-natal facilities and screening for cervical and breast cancer. Working-class people are more likely to live in inner-city areas, where standards of general practice, which includes an important element of health education and preventive medicine, are inadequate. They are less able to bypass waiting lists for "non-urgent" operations such as prostatectomy and hip replacement by using private medicine. Tudor-Hart (1971) has summed up these class gradients in health as the *inverse care law,* which states that good medical care is *least* likely to be available to those who are *most* in need of it.

This evidence on the quality and distribution of medical care has important implications for psychotherapy. Although, in the United Kingdom, working-class people visit their family doctors and use hospital services more than do the middle class, the care they receive, from the psychotherapeutic point of view, is likely to be inferior. A working-class patient presenting to a doctor with emotional distress is likely to be prescribed a tranquillizer. Middle-class patients are more likely to see a doctor who offers simple psychotherapy, rather than a prescription. Tranquillizers are often a token currency of heteronomous dependency which inhibits change; psychotherapeutic dependency, on the other hand, can be a precursor to greater understanding and autonomy. On the face of it, it does not seem fair that distressed working-class people should be tranquillized while their middle-class counterparts are more likely to receive psychotherapy.

Tyrill Harris and George Brown's well-known studies on depression provide support for the view that there is, proportionally, a greater need for psychotherapy among working-class women (Brown & Harris, 1978). They found that in the Camberwell district of southeast London depression was four times commoner among working-class than among middle-class women. Since there is a strong link between depression and loss, the researchers thought at first that the class difference might be due entirely to the increased incidence of painful loss-events in the lives of working-class women. For example, they and their families are more likely to experience unemployment, redundancy, homelessness, bereavement, and difficulties with school and the law. While all this was true, it accounted for only a minor part of the class difference in depression rates. Harris and Brown showed that it is not just loss itself that is linked to depression, but *loss in a particular context.* Where women are well supported by a spouse or companion in whom they can confide, they are more able to withstand loss without developing depression.

For Harris and Brown, *self-esteem* was the key to the problems that they were investigating, and to their solution. Adverse conditions of life, especially loss and bereavement, erode self-esteem; good relationships and a feeling of effectiveness enhance it. Autonomy and self-esteem are very closely connected. Lack of control over one's life, and lack of understanding as to how that lack of control has come about, create a chronic spiral of heteronomy. A feeling of effectiveness, of control, of being able to form good relationships, of having some understanding of the reasons for and limits to areas that are beyond one's control, all contribute to a sense of autonomy. Becoming autonomous is likely to lead to self-esteem and the benign circles of health; enhanced self-esteem gives one the courage and acceptance to become more autonomous.

Psychotherapy enhances both self-esteem and autonomy. It provides the kind of intimate, confiding relationship that Harris and Brown found was lacking in depressed women. It increases self-knowledge and enables grief to be accepted rather than suppressed. It provides the support and encouragement that are needed for people to undertake effective action. Given that this is so, the increased suffering and the decreased buffering that apply to working-class people means that there is a *prima facie* case for making psychotherapy more rather than less available to them compared with their middle-class counterparts.

The evidence suggests that the reverse is the case. Hollingshead and Redlich's (1958) classic study, originally published in 1954, showed that in the United States it was class rather than need or diagnosis that was the key determinant of the type of psychiatric treatment that a patient received: social classes I and II received psychotherapy, whereas classes IV and V received drugs and electroconvulsive therapy. Follow-up studies published thirty years later show that the overall pattern has not changed greatly (Mollica & Milic, 1986).

If, as we argued in chapter three, autonomy is a basic need rather than a luxury, then this inequality in access to psychotherapy appears to be a serious inequity. And, as we discuss further in chapter five, in suggesting that psychotherapy provision for working-class people needs to be increased, we are not, Marie-Antoinette-like, merely offering a non-essential—and for that matter, non-existent—cake because there is no bread.

We are claiming that the class differential in psychiatric morbidity strongly suggests that large numbers of working-class people are likely to need a considerable amount of psychotherapy. Yet it is by no means clear that this is what they *want*. Is, then, our proposal for the expansion of psychotherapy not just a disguised form of authoritarian paternalism? We think not, for two reasons. First, we are not suggesting that psychotherapy be imposed on unwilling recipients. Second, the needs we speak of are actually grounded in genuine wants. We believe that the sorts of benefits offered by psychotherapy, such as improved self-esteem, improved relationships, and greater emotional autonomy, are either wanted by nearly everyone or, if not wanted, are necessary conditions for things that are wanted.

To meet these needs, psychotherapy has to become both much more widely *available,* and much more *accessible* to those who need it. Any programme for the expansion of psychotherapy should, as we discuss, take these points into account. But first we look at how the unequal distribution of psychotherapy comes about.

How the needy are denied psychotherapy

There are several obstacles that a patient in search of psychotherapy, especially if it is to be provided by the state, must negotiate before treatment is achieved. These act as barriers progressively reducing the numbers of working-class patients who are taken on. There are three main types of barrier: geographical and financial obstacles; selection bias; and conflict of expectations, arising largely out of psychotherapeutic technique.

Geographical and financial obstacles

Many people are denied access both to state and private psycho-therapy simply by reason of geography. There is a huge pull towards the metropolis. The British Psychoanalytic Society has some 400 members and associate members; of these the vast majority live and work in London and its suburbs. In 1997, there were about 130 consultant psychotherapists working within the British National Health Services; of these, about 70 work in London and the southeast. The Tavistock Institute, the main centre for psychotherapy training in the NHS, which is nationally funded, is located in London: it takes 90 per cent of its patients and 70 per cent of its trainees from the southeast, although it does make strenuous efforts to reach out to the remoter parts of the country. Even allowing for the fact that one-third of the population of the United Kingdom lives in the southeast, the disproportion is startling. Those regions that are least affluent—and, if the Black Report is correct, are likely to have the *highest* mental illness rates—have the *least adequate* psychotherapy provision.

Inequality in publicly funded psychotherapy could in theory, though not so easily in practice, as we shall see shortly, be redressed by greatly increasing psychotherapy resources in the provinces.

In the United Kingdom psychotherapy is one of the most privatized sectors of recognized health care, and the cost of private psychotherapy puts it beyond the reach of many working-class people. Even those with private health insurance may be unable to pay for it since psychotherapy is not covered by many insurance policies. Nine months of once-weekly therapy, which many would consider a modest course of treatment, might cost around £1,000. This is not, it might be argued, an extraordinary amount when set, say, against the cost of a foreign holiday or a new car, but it is a lot for someone to have to pay for essential health care. And, as we have argued, many of those who are most in need of psychotherapy are often the least able to afford holidays, cars, or health care.

Selection bias for state-funded psychotherapy

Despite financial and geographical obstacles to an equitable distribution of psychotherapeutic care, publicly funded psychotherapy *does* exist, and one might expect that, once referred, working-class patients would have an equal chance of receiving and benefiting from treatment. In fact this is not so. Numerous studies, mostly from the United States, have shown a subtle class bias influencing both referral and *selection* for state-funded psychotherapy (Lorion & Felner, 1986). Two British studies also suggest that the bias operates in the United Kingdom.

Lorna and John Wing studied a psychiatric training institute that accepted referrals from far away but also had a small adjacent catchment area (Wing & Wing, 1970). Their study revealed that those offered psychotherapy tended to be non-catchment area middle-class patients, while working-class catchment area patients, despite comparable diagnoses, received drugs and other non-psychotherapeutic treatments. Similar conclusions emerged from Holmes's study of selection for psychotherapy in an inner-city group practice in London (Holmes, 1987). Although the practice had a strong tradition of concern for the disadvantaged, bias against working-class patients was found to be operating at several levels. Only 40 per cent of patients referred by GPs for psychotherapy were working class, rather than the 60 to 70 per cent that would be expected from the class composition of the practice. Further selection occurred after assessment by the consultant psychotherapist. Only 27 per cent of those considered suitable for formal psychotherapy were working class, and only 14 per cent of those taken on by experienced, as opposed to trainee, psychotherapists were working class. In considering psychotherapy for working-class people, it seems that few are called, and fewer still are chosen.

One frequently given reason for this bias against selecting working-class patients is that middle-class people are consistently seen as more motivated, more likely to benefit from, and therefore more attractive patients for psychotherapy. If these perceptions are accurate, is it not right that the bias should operate? What is the point of offering inappropriate treatment to people who are unlikely to benefit from it? Could it not be argued that, although unequal, selection for psychotherapy is not inequitable?

State-funded psychotherapy is a rare commodity, so selection for it should be rigorous. Irrespective of class, only about half of those referred are taken on for psychotherapy. With the scarcity of state-funded psychotherapists, it is particularly important that their time should not be wasted on those who are unlikely to benefit, and particularly on those who are likely to drop out of treatment before it has had a chance to be effective.

Several studies have shown that drop-out rates are consistently highest among working-class patients. In one study, only 12 per cent of working-class patients remained in treatment for thirty sessions compared with 42 per cent of middle-class patients. In another, there was "a clear linear relationship between social class and continuation in psychotherapy, with increasing proportions of drop-outs as social class level decreased. The range was from zero in Class I to 50 per cent in Class V" (Garfield, 1986). Inequalities in selection for psychotherapy can be justified by citing evidence such as this. However, in asking whether present practice is *morally* acceptable, and whether something ought to be done to change it, we need to look at some of the reasons why working-class patients are relatively likely to drop out of psychotherapy, even if therapy is available for them and they have been offered it.

Conflict of expectations

An important reason for the high drop-out rate among working-class patients arises from a conflict of expectations. Analytic psychotherapists usually view therapy as a prolonged treatment lasting for months at least, with only a gradual resolution of problems. It has been shown that working-class patients, who often drop out after four to six sessions, expect therapy to be brief and problems to be solved quickly, with more advice, reassurance, and direction than most therapists would expect to offer (Lorion & Felner, 1986).

It is likely that several aspects of psychotherapeutic technique are off-putting to working-class patients, and there is good evidence that where technique is modified drop-out rates are lower (Heitler, 1976). Patients who have preparatory pre-treatment sessions explaining what psychotherapy is about drop out less, and have better outcomes than those who have no such explanation; combining drug and psychotherapeutic treatment in depressed women produces fewer working-class drop-outs; brief therapy gives better results with working-class patients than open-ended treatment.

In chapter one we mentioned the three elements of psychotherapy: structure, space for exploration, and the therapeutic relationship itself. Given the present organization and construction of psychotherapy, each of these is likely to work to the relative disadvantage of working-class patients.

Structure

Formal psychotherapy requires regular meetings at a place and time usually chosen by and convenient for the therapist.

TWO PATIENTS WHO HAD DIFFICULTY WITH TIME

A working-class patient arrived exactly one hour late for her assessment interview, just as the therapist was about to collect his next patient. The patient explained that she always arrived an hour late for hospital appointments since she had found this reduced the average waiting time to see the consultant to about half an hour! Another patient, who was well motivated and suitable for therapy, insisted that she could manage appointments only after 5 p.m. She worked as a tea lady on a building site and could not get away before then. In a middle-class patient, with more opportunities for flexible organization of time, such an insistence might well have been a defence against therapy (saying she wanted it, but really being reluctant to commit herself). For this working-class patient, it was an inescapable reality.

An underlying assumption of most psychotherapy is that, as Epictetus put it, "men are troubled not by things, but their appreciation of things". Psychotherapists may be unaware of how difficult it is for working-class patients to detach themselves sufficiently from "things", including the struggle to survive, sufficiently to pursue a course of psychotherapy.

Elements of frustration are intrinsic to therapy. Short-term solutions to problems are rarely offered. If the problem is located within the individual's personality, a premature reaching for "solutions" may be an avoidance of the growth that is needed before the problem can be effectively tackled. The analytic therapist resists enacting the roles of friend, comforter, guide, and support in which the patient casts her. These transferential projections are, as we discuss in chapter six, eventually handed back to be reintegrated into the patient's personality, and so enhance autonomy.

But this technical approach is predicated on the assumption that a patient's distress is primarily psychological, and that the environment, if properly approached, will not be too hostile and thwarting but will eventually yield to the individual's more realistic desires. One psychotherapist described the typical patient seeking publicly funded psychotherapy as "middle class with delusions of poverty" (N. Symington, personal communication, 1980). As Epstein (1995) argues, when poverty is *not* a delusion psychotherapy becomes more problematic.

Space for exploration of feelings

Psychotherapy patients are invited and expected to explore their feelings primarily through language. Bernstein's classic study of language and psychotherapy distinguishes between "restrictive" and "elaborated" codes of language (Bernstein, 1964). The study claims that working-class people are more likely to use the former, middle-class the latter. Working-class patients may find psychotherapeutic exploration of feelings and fantasies more difficult than middle-class

patients, since these explorations are usually pursued through elaborated codes of language. This study can be criticized on the grounds
that the researchers, themselves middle class, were insensitive to the
elaborations of working-class language, but it is still very relevant to
psychotherapy. The intimidating silence of the therapy session in
which the patient is encouraged to "explore her feelings" can easily
be experienced by patients, especially if working class, as self-indul-
gent or persecutory. Whether or not the patient would be able under
different circumstances to explore her feelings, such a technique,
particularly if not properly explained, is likely to lead to drop-out or
to an assessment of unsuitability.

Therapeutic relationship (identification)

Identification between patient and therapist is an essential ingredient of psychotherapy. The patient has to feel that whatever
differences of age, sex, colour, culture, experience, and values exist
between patient and therapist, these are outweighed by a common
humanity. This is the basis of empathy, without which successful
therapy is impossible.

Our discussion in this chapter has so far focused on class-based
barriers and biases in psychotherapy. Equally important issues are
raised by questions of *gender* and sexism in psychotherapy: these
include the theoretical bias in the classical Freudian view of female
psychology; the exploitation and even seduction of female patients by
male therapists (see chapter eight); and the possible invalidation of
legitimate feminist social aims by a patriarchal psychotherapeutic
ethic.

Although the majority of therapists and patients are probably
women, senior positions, as in other professions, tend to be occupied
by men. Senior analysts and other therapists—like university profes-
sors as opposed to primary school teachers—are, more often than not,
white males, middle class in background, experience, and outlook.
This might well make identification more difficult between senior
and therefore opinion-forming therapists and black, female, or working-class patients. It is hardly surprising, given the nature of the
therapeutic relationship, that the majority of therapists would see
middle-class patients with similar experiences and outlooks to their
own as more attractive for therapy than working-class patients.

Equally, it may be difficult for a poor, unemployed, or intimidated patient to identify with the obviously affluent therapist in a comfortable job and at home in the institution that is offering therapy.

This issue is well illustrated by the following description by the feminist therapist Sheila Ernst of her difficulties in "identification" with a therapist whose experiences, way of life, and values seemed very different from her own:

> My analyst wore a suit, lived in a large house in a middle class suburb with a neat garden, had a wife who didn't work and a spotless child who went to private school. I still don't know what his assumptions were about women's role or what he thought about my attempts to combine being a student with taking most of the responsibility for the house and my small step-son, and being a trade union activist. . . . He was not oppressive in the blatant way that feminist writers on therapy have documented. He didn't try to seduce me, tell me I should use make-up or dress differently, accuse me of being incapable of real love because I didn't have orgasms. . . . The oppression lay in *who he was*, the questions *he didn't ask* and the material *I didn't present*. It lay in the way I felt when I arrived at his house on my bicycle and he drew up in his large car; in the sense that I had that he must see his wife and family and home as normal and my household as a sign of my abnormality. To be cured would be to be capable of living like him. [Ernst & Goodison, 1981]

An example such as this raises important technical as well as ethical questions. Does this difference of values between Ernst and her therapist matter, or could he still be a technically good therapist for her, despite the age and gender gap? Was there really a class barrier, or was the student Ernst suffering from "delusions of poverty"? Could these feelings not have come up for productive discussion and exploration in the therapy?

We would answer these and related questions along two main lines. First, within any therapeutic relationship there are bound to be differences of values, attitude, and taste. These are not necessarily a barrier to successful therapy, because the aim is to help the patient autonomously to find her own values and choices, not to impose those of the therapist. The inevitable discrepancies in outlook and position between therapist and patient *can* be used productively in therapy if they are understood in terms of transference—that is, the expectations, hopes, and desires that the patient projects onto the therapist and the differences between these and reality. Freud saw neurosis as a "turning away from reality". Psychotherapy can help people to face up to reality, which is a pre-condition of changing it. But there is clearly a danger that transference interpretations of real differences will be used by the therapist to distance himself from and deny difficulties about contrasts between his own and the patient's social position.

This leads to our second answer to the questions raised by Ernst's difficulties, which will form the focus of the remainder of this chapter. If it is true that many potential patients are deterred by the apparent elitism of many therapists, then psychotherapy, if it is to address the real issue of injustice and not remain a preserve for the privileged few, must be prepared to modify and broaden its attitudes and techniques.

Attitudes

In her book *Therapy in the Ghetto*, Lerner (1972) reported on a five-year project on analytic psychotherapy with working-class patients. Forty-five patients suffering from depression and anxiety were seen by fifteen different therapists for an average of about twenty sessions each. Twelve patients dropped out, but twenty-six of the thirty-three who stayed on showed marked improvement. Lerner found a significant association between therapists who had a "democratic attitude" and patient improvement. The research required an assessment of the extent to which the therapist saw working-class patients as having equal value, potential, and creativity to middle-class patients. As Lerner puts it, democratic, non-authoritarian attitudes "create an ambience in which clients avail themselves of their own resources [and] . . . make it easier for very confused and needy people to avail themselves of other good things the therapist has to offer, such as warmth, acceptance, protection, understanding and clarification" (Lerner, 1972).

Would-be psychotherapeutic democrats must offer more than warmth and acceptance, however, as the next example shows. No matter how hard therapists try to be less remote and elitist, there are bound to be real differences in power, status, security, and income between them and their poorer patients, which cannot be glossed over by charitable attitudes.

THE MAN WHO COULD NOT TRUST

A young man was being seen for supportive psychotherapy. He had been brought up in the East End of London in conditions of emotional and material poverty. After leaving school, he worked for a while in printing firm. When he was 18 his mother died of cancer. He became very depressed, gave up work, and refused to leave the house where he lived with his father, who was a cantankerous respiratory cripple. A visiting psychiatrist diagnosed schizophrenia, probably wrongly, and prescribed monthly injections of a major tranquillizer. The young man continued with these for three years, but remained confined to his house. One day he had a violent row with his father, and left to live in another part of the city. Through the Social Services Department he was housed in a bed and breakfast hotel, and eventually referred again for psychiatric help because of his obvious depression. As his therapist got to know him, it became clear that his whole world view was based on mistrust and suspicion. "How can you expect me to trust anyone?" he ranted. His father was a "bastard", the psychiatrist who gave him the injections "ought to be locked up", the social workers were "no good " and kept offering him flats that were "useless": everyone let him down, kept him waiting, didn't care.

The therapist listened patiently to these tirades, and at first had no difficulty in empathizing with his plight. He tried, unsuccessfully, to steer the patient's thoughts to his mother's death and the anger and disappointment that it had left him with. Feeling that the patient needed more than he could offer, he suggested that it might be helpful if the patient were to attend a day hospital. The patient suddenly became furious. "How can you make suggestions like that?" he shouted. "You don't realize how difficult it is for me to come here to the hospital, let alone go into a new situation with strangers. " The therapist replied that perhaps he felt he was being passed on or got rid of, just as he may have felt abandoned when his mother died. Perhaps this was what had made him so angry. The patient lost his temper: "You middle-class bastard, you don't give a damn about me, sitting there with your well-paid job, your nice wife and kids, and comfortable home in the suburbs. What do the likes of you know about the way I live—

in a damp room with no money, noisy neighbours, no job, walking the streets in the freezing cold?" [It was a wintry November day.] "You're just doing your job, waiting to go home, you don't care about me one bit."

The force of this outburst was shocking. The attack had hit home, leaving the therapist speechless and inadequate. In the end he replied that while he accepted the validity of what the patient had said, he also felt that the patient was using his misery in a self-destructive way. The patient's no doubt accurate perception of his therapist's concerns for his own life should not be a justification for inertia, or become a way of avoiding the need to find a future and to free himself from a paralysing attachment to his dead mother. The patient missed the next two sessions, but, rather to the therapist's surprise, did return, and work continued. Eventually the patient attended the day hospital and, while remaining on the fringes of "normal" society, became less depressed and paranoid.

It is no doubt desirable for therapists to adopt a democratic attitude towards their patients. At the same time, the containing therapeutic "frame" must be maintained. Langs has suggested that the apparent failure of analytic therapy with poor patients results from patronizing "frame violation" on the part of the therapist (Cheifetz, 1984). Here the patient reacted furiously to the possible frame-breaking rejection. The example shows, too, how effective therapy may require an acknowledgement, rather than avoidance, of the inequalities between therapist and patient. Justice does not require the elimination of all differences between people, but rather the eradication of arbitrary disadvantage. Many arbitrary disadvantages are caused by factors that psychotherapy, by its nature, cannot change (see chapter five). One of its key functions is to help patients overcome psychological barriers that prevent awareness of the full reality of their situation, so that they can change what needs to be changed and perhaps adapt to what cannot be changed. Yet psychotherapy remains unavailable or inaccessible to many disadvantaged people whose need for it is great. This inequity is something that psychotherapists could, and should, address.

Attempts to overcome class bias in psychotherapy

If the distribution of psychotherapy *is* unfair, what ought to be done about it? In order to answer this, we look at attempts that have been made to overcome class bias in psychotherapy and consider some more radical approaches to the problem of bridging the gap between ordinary people and the rarefied world of psychotherapy. It should be noted at this point that similar concerns have been raised about racial bias in psychotherapy, especially where it overlaps with class, since to be black often means to be economically disadvantaged as well (D. Holmes, 1992). There are three main ways in which attempts have been made to overcome class bias in psychotherapy: by widening its availability, by targeting, and by modification of technique.

Widening the availability of psychotherapy

Hollingshead and Redlich showed how working-class patients in the United States were denied access to psychotherapy (Hollingshead & Redlich, 1958). In the liberal atmosphere of the late 1960s and early 1970s, there was a proliferation of community mental health centres throughout the United States, which aimed to bring analytic psychotherapy to the poor and deprived.

Evaluative studies of the Community Mental Health Movement have revealed mixed results (Mollica & Milic, 1986). Working-class patients with neurotic disorders are now somewhat more likely to be offered psychotherapy than they were, but the unemployed, especially men, continue to be seriously under-represented among those who are offered psychotherapy as opposed to merely physical methods of treatment. The drop-out rate among working-class patients remains very high. In most settings few working-class patients receive more than six sessions of therapy.

In the United Kingdom, the NHS and the highly developed social services network should in theory be an ideal vehicle for making psychotherapy generally available. There has been some expansion of specialized psychotherapy within the NHS. The first consultant psychotherapist was appointed in 1964, and there are now about a hundred such posts. There is a need for a further expansion in the number of consultant psychotherapists, but this in itself would not *guarantee* that less well-off patients would achieve greater access to psychotherapy.

There is an analogy with the expansion of higher education that took place in Britain in the 1960s and 1970s following the Robbins Report. The Report recommended that higher education should be made available to all those seeking and able to benefit from it. As a result, the total *number* of students from working-class homes entering university went up, but the *proportion* of students with a working-class background has not significantly increased.

One possible reason for this relative exclusion of working-class patients is that psychotherapy has been dominated by the ethos of what might be called "high-culture" psychotherapy, which is predominantly psychoanalytic and, although well suited for educated middle-class professionals, may be less appropriate for others.

To continue the comparison with post-secondary education: "high-culture" psychotherapy might be likened to the educational role of Oxford and Cambridge at the end of the nineteenth century before the educational franchise was widened. Early attempts to bring psychotherapy out of its ivory tower failed because unmodified psychoanalytic attitudes and techniques, while quite appropriate in their own context, do not take when transplanted into the less privileged and more pressurized world beyond.

Simply widening the availability of analytic psychotherapy, while laudable and necessary, is insufficient to achieve the goal of seeing that working-class people receive psychotherapy when they need it.

Targeting

One promising approach is to concentrate psychotherapy resources on particular target groups and locations. The setting up of women's therapy centres is a good example. These have been very successful in attracting into therapy working-class women who might otherwise be put off by the psychological and practical barriers surrounding conventional psychotherapy departments. Targeting of this sort has the additional advantage of encouraging therapists to develop theoretical and technical approaches that are especially relevant to the group in question. Similar centres have been established, although many more are needed, offering counselling and psychotherapy to ethnic minorities. Therapy services based in general practice, on housing estates, in child health clinics, and in factories, schools, and colleges are all extensions of the idea that psychotherapy should be brought to the people.

Targeting can, however, be problematic. As a welfare strategy it runs the danger of creating a two-tier system, with well-funded, often private, therapy for the middle classes, and a shoe-string second-class service for the less well-off. Therapists working in "target" settings can become socially and intellectually isolated. Much stronger links and interchanges are needed between the psychoanalytic establishment and the newer (less "high-culture") therapies. Each needs to learn from the other and modify its ideas and practice accordingly.

Changing techniques

Freud realized the need for modifications of technique when he wrote:

> One may reasonably expect that at some time or other the conscience of the community will awake and admonish it that the poor man has just as much right to help for his mind as he now has for the surgeon's means for saving his life . . . the task will then arise for us to adapt our techniques to the new conditions. I have no doubt that we shall need to find the simplest and most natural expression for our theoretical doctrines. [Freud, 1919a]

In a much-quoted passage he wrote of "alloying the pure gold of psychoanalysis with the baser metals of suggestion". He thought that psychoanalytic technique would have to be modified if its benefits were to extend beyond the middle-class intelligentsia. We have already described ways in which "high-culture" psychoanalysis is unsuitable for large numbers of people who need therapy. We now briefly describe how therapeutic technique may be modified so as to make it more accessible; we also point out some of the inherent difficulties in trying to "bring psychotherapy to the people".

Brief dynamic psychotherapy

Brief psychotherapy arose out of the need to find a form of analytic psychotherapy that would be appropriate for people from a wide range of backgrounds, could be applicable within state-funded settings such as the NHS, and yet remain true to the principles of psychoanalysis.

In the United Kingdom, brief psychotherapy was pioneered by David Malan at the Tavistock Clinic (Malan, 1963). As well as being, as its name suggests, limited in time, brief psychotherapy has other features that make it more accessible to working-class patients. It is focused, and to some extent goal-directed; the therapist assumes an active, guiding role; and the patient is given a clearer view of what is likely to happen and what is expected of her. On the other hand, Malan advocates a strict selection procedure for brief psychotherapy, which has the effect of favouring middle-class patients in a number of ways.

Certain categories of patient are excluded: namely, the suicidal and those actively abusing drugs or alcohol. This counts against working-class patients, who, for cultural as well as intrapsychic reasons, are more likely to manifest disturbance in these ways.

Brief psychotherapy is not considered suitable for very disturbed patients. Middle-class patients are more likely than working-class patients to be referred for specialist treatment before they are severely ill. This is true for medical referrals in general, not just for those concerning psychological disorders. As a result, proportionately fewer suitable working-class patients are available for brief psychotherapy.

A third problem is that an important selection factor for brief psychotherapy is the capacity of the patient to show in the assessment interview that she can "work in the transference", in other words, express and understand feelings towards the therapist. This leads to precisely the difficulties for working-class patients that we pointed out in our discussion of selection.

Despite the development of a therapy that has considerable potential for benefiting less advantaged patients, there are thus powerful forces that exclude them and favour middle-class people. These must be taken into account in planning a more equitable psychotherapy service.

Behavioural and cognitive behavioural psychotherapies

As discussed in chapter two, the development of cognitive behaviour therapy (CBT), with its emphasis on thought patterns as well as actions, and the adoption of a more active role by analytic therapists in brief therapy, have narrowed the gap between analytic and behavioural psychotherapies. CBT has become a very popular form of therapy, with a wide range of applicability, especially in anxiety-based disorders and in depression. Its possible use in helping psychotic patients to live more comfortably with their delusions is another recent application which is being actively researched. There is preliminary evidence that young psychotic males from ethnic minorities—who previously would have been considered totally unsuitable for psychotherapy—can be helped by this approach, and their use of psychotropic drugs can be much reduced as a result (Chadwick & Birchwood, 1994).

Behaviour therapy is brief and symptom-focused, with declared goals. Behaviour therapists can be trained in a comparatively short time, and a successful targeting strategy has meant that many nurses trained in behaviour therapy are now attached to general practices. All this means that behaviour therapy is far more equitably distributed than analytic therapy.

However, if emotional autonomy is the principal goal of psychotherapy, the immediacy and symptom focus of behaviour therapy can also be a limitation, as the following example illustrates.

THE WOMAN WHO COULD NOT GO OUT

A middle-aged woman with agoraphobic symptoms became entirely reliant on her husband because of her inability to leave the house. She was helped by behaviour therapy offered by a community nurse. But her dependency was then transferred to this therapist, a warm, good-looking young man, and not long after the sessions stopped her symptoms returned. Subsequent, more analytically oriented, sessions explored her boredom, unexpressed anger with her husband, and difficulty in accepting her separation from her daughter when she left home to get married. As a child she had had to look after her mother who suffered from multiple sclerosis and with whom, through the "handling" of her agoraphobia, she had partially identified. The feelings of grief, guilt, and anger that this left her with, and the way in which she had re-enacted them through her own "illness", were not tackled by the exclusively symptom-oriented approach of the initial behavioural sessions.

Behavioural and cognitive behavioural therapies form a vital part of a more equitable psychotherapy service. When combined with, and sometimes leading on to, more analytically oriented treatment, they have the potential for an important liberating effect that goes far beyond symptom removal.

Family and marital therapy

The emergence of family and marital therapy as a major therapeutic mode has been an important development in psychotherapy. Its potential for benefiting working-class patients was demonstrated in the 1960s in the former psychoanalyst Salvador Minuchin's classic study *Families of the Slums* (Minuchin et al., 1963), in which he showed that delinquent ghetto children became less disturbed, and not merely more conformist, in response to family therapy.

From the point of view of working-class patients, family therapy lacks many of the drawbacks of analytic therapies. It is usually brief and directive, with a strong behavioural component. It is useful in a wide range of conditions and is not limited by the age or educational level of the patient. As we mentioned in chapter two, important recent research has shown that family intervention can prevent relapse in schizophrenia.

Working-class patients may also be more likely to experience a problem in terms of a rift within the family, rather than locating it within themselves as individuals. Exploring, clarifying, or healing that rift makes immediate sense. The problems associated with working-class patients feeling overwhelmed and intimidated by therapists are also less serious in family therapy, which works from strengths rather than from weaknesses (Holmes, 1985). A working-class patient who, at an individual level, might find it hard to form a therapeutic relationship with an analytic therapist may, in a family context, gain strength and solidarity which, if internalized, will enhance self-esteem.

* * *

This rather abbreviated discussion of brief, behavioural, and family and marital therapies bears out the view, put forward in chapter two, that no *one* form of psychotherapy can claim special status. We are arguing here that, for psychotherapy to cater more fairly for the needs of patients, a much broader range of therapy options must be available than the purely analytic.

We have suggested that there may indeed be special features of analytic therapy which, in a stratified society, make it unattractive and unsuitable for the worst-off. Without symptom alleviation, autonomy is impossible, and for working-class patients in particular, relief from symptoms may be an immediate priority. At the same time, analytic therapy, with its emphasis on understanding which goes beyond symptom removal, is especially important because of its capacity to enhance emotional autonomy. There remains a need to find forms of therapy that raise consciousness and enhance autonomy in the way that psychoanalysis can, without being so exclusive and elitist. The potential conflict between the need for relief and the need for autonomy was apparent to some of the early psychoanalytic pioneers, notably Sandor Ferenczi, who emphasized the importance of "active emotional experience" as opposed to merely intellectual understanding in therapy (Ferenczi, 1960), and Wilhelm Reich, who attempted to combine Marxist and psychoanalytic perspectives (Reich, 1961). It is to the legacy of some of their ideas that we now turn.

Humanistic psychology and psycho-politics

Since the origins of the psychoanalytic movement, there has been a tension between psychotherapy and politics. A radical political critic of those who have attempted to modify therapeutic techniques in the ways we have just been discussing could argue that they are just tinkering with the problem. There is no chance of providing an adequate psychotherapeutic service until the fundamental material inequalities between people have been tackled. On the other hand, a psychotherapist aware of the connection between an inequitable psychotherapy service and a more broadly unjust society could reply that it is unlikely that a better society will arise unless the people within it can be personally changed for the better, and that psychotherapy may contribute significantly to producing that change. The tension between psychotherapy and politics is well expressed by Bruno Bettelheim, describing his personal experience of intellectual struggle as an adolescent growing up in inter-war Austria among the assimilated Jewish bourgeoisie:

> In order to create the good society, was it of first importance to change society radically enough for all persons to achieve full

self-realisation? In this case psychoanalysis could be discarded, with the possible exception of a few deranged persons. Or was this the wrong approach, and could only persons who had achieved full personal liberation and integration by being psychoanalysed create such a "good" society? In the latter case the correct thing was to forget for the time being any social or economic revolution and to concentrate instead on pushing psychoanalysis; the hope was that once the vast majority of men had profited from its inner liberation they would almost automatically create the good society for themselves and all others. [Bettelheim, 1960]

The post-war years saw a series of historical developments and cultural shifts that combined to alter the terms of Bettelheim's dilemma. These included the re-discovery in the 1950s of Marx's *Economic and Philosophical Manuscripts* with their emphasis on personal as well as political liberation; the growth of the feminist movement, which has linked the individual and psychological problems of women to their social position; and the increasing emphasis on a cultural as well as an economic critique of Western social structures. These developments led to the establishment of "humanistic psychology", with an emphasis on *experience* rather than *thought*; attempts to demystify therapy by self-help therapies such as co-counselling, where participants exchange roles of therapist and patient with each other; and attempts to break through directly to repressed feelings and forgotten memories through "encounter groups" and psychodrama. All these underlie renewed attempts to produce a therapeutic ("psy-pol") movement that would overcome both the traditional psychoanalytic detachment from political and social reality and the blindness of conventional polities to psychology. Its theoretical expression has been summarized in these terms:

> There are in fact many striking parallels between the work of a psychotherapist and the work of a political activist. One could say that each is involved in a form of "consciousness raising". Both the therapist and the political actor seeks to be emancipatory. Just as the therapist seeks to assist the individual to obtain some degree of emancipation from the intangible private inner forces to which so much of his or her life is a reaction, so does the political actor seek to enable classes and other social formations to act upon, rather than react to, intangible public forces. [Hogget & Lonsada, 1985]

As we mention in chapter eleven, the shift in modern polities towards more pluralistic, individualistic approaches provides opportunities for further parallels between personal and social emancipation. Samuels (1993) has argued that there has been a repression of the "political psyche"—the part of the mind that is concerned with power relations between the self and society—and has developed a method of group discussion whose objective is to help people get in touch with this aspect of themselves and so become more involved in the politics of their everyday lives. Some psychotherapists are beginning to argue that public life is often devoid of psychological insight, and that politicians and policymakers could benefit from understanding the psychological impact of their behaviour and policies (see, for example, Kraemer & Roberts, 1996).

"Community psychotherapy"

Humanistic psychology can, however, be no less of a middle-class preserve than analytic psychotherapy, and the quest for personal liberation an avoidance of, rather than a first step towards, addressing the real inequities of a divided society (see chapter five). Nevertheless the "psy-pol" approach has led to a number of important projects in deprived inner-city areas, which attempt simultaneously to address the material problems of the *community* and the psychological difficulties of its members, especially women (Holland & Holland, 1984). They aim to combat a number of material difficulties such as poor housing, poverty, and lack of child-care facilities, and at the same time to link these with and help overcome psychological difficulties such as lack of assertiveness, inability to express anger in constructive ways, poor marital and sexual relationships, difficulties with child-rearing, and tranquillizer dependency.

The community psychotherapist has the role of a social catalyst fostering self-help links between the isolated and deprived, helping those who are politically active to attempt also to overcome psychological difficulties, and to see how political activity can be a diversion from these, and helping others to use their new-found strengths of assertiveness and creative anger to alter not just their relationships but their material circumstances.

Although these projects have yet to be fully evaluated, and often depend for their success on a fortunate mix of charismatic yet democratic leadership from the psychotherapist and receptiveness in the community, they are examples of what can be achieved, and it is likely that they have had influence far beyond the particular housing estates or run-down streets that they serve. The principles of targeting psychological services in a deprived area, of self-help groups, and of a flexible focus on both material and psychological difficulties are all steps towards achieving a more egalitarian psychotherapy service. The attachment of counsellors and psychotherapists to general practice, training psychotherapists who do not necessarily have conventional educational qualifications, and the use of housing or health issues as starting points for psychological enquiry are promising examples of such developments.

Psychoanalysis and democratic psychotherapy

For community psychotherapy to remain psychotherapeutic as well as communal, it will need to maintain strong links with the central body of analytic ideas and practice. Sadly, the response of the psychoanalytic establishment to attempts to bring psychotherapy closer to ordinary people has not always been positive. Psychoanalysts have remained a closed group, at times almost a secret society. They defend their rigorous selection and training procedures, and counter any charges of elitism with the argument that anything less than the full-blown analytic approach, even if it does exclude the majority of ordinary people, requires an intolerable watering down of the unique methods and insights of psychoanalysis. No doubt there is validity in this, but it can appear as a defensive reaction to the threat posed by the flowering of non-analytic therapies which has taken place over the past decade.

In response to the charge of inequity, the psychoanalytic establishment tends to fall back on Freud's dictum that the essence of psychoanalysis is not *therapy*, of which there are many forms, but a unique way of reaching the *truth*. Any treatment that compromises on the pursuit of truth is bound to be seen as defective. This purist argument runs the risk of reducing the importance that psychoanalysis could have in a psychotherapy profession that catered properly for patients' needs.

Rather than addressing the question of elitism, some psychoanalysts have instead tried to "interpret" the criticisms of those who claim that psychoanalysis is elitist and inequitable, and effectively to question their motivation in so doing. There are interesting parallels here with the defensiveness of psychoanalysts in the face of the criticism that their methods are not scientific, which we discussed in chapter two.

These psychoanalysts regard "community psychotherapy" as a kind of prostitution: they claim that the "monogamy" of analyst and analysed cannot be shared out in this way without destroying its essence; they argue that ignoble impulses like envy and greed, which psychoanalysis alone has the power to unveil, are perpetuated by phoney democratization rather than transcended by understanding.

This rather depressing, though no doubt not completely implausible, argument is taken a stage further by the distinguished French psychoanalyst Janine Chasseguet-Smirgel. She likens the levelling-down wish (in this context, the desire to modify therapy so that it fits the needs and expectations of working-class people) to a perversion. She sees it as a denial of reality, of the real differences between people; in her terms, the "double difference", the difference between generations and the difference between the sexes. This perverse solution is a "balm for our wounded narcissism and a means of dissipating our feelings of smallness and inadequacy. This temptation can lead to our losing the love of truth and replacing it with a taste for sham" (Chasseguet-Smirgel, 1985).

According to her, preoccupation with poverty, with dirt, is part of a general regression in which authority and leadership are denied. She connects the psychological celebration of sadism by de Sade with the politics of the French Revolution. The origins of this, according to Chasseguet-Smirgel, lie in the wish to escape the "paternal order":

> The pervert will attempt to give himself and others the illusion that anal sexuality (which is accessible to the little boy) is equal and even superior to genital sexuality (accessible to the father). . . . In reality, in order to have a genital penis and to procreate, it is necessary to grow up, to mature, to wait, whereas faeces are a production common to adult and child, woman and man. The two differences between the sexes and between generations are abolished at the anal level. Time is wiped out. [Chasseguet-Smirgel, 1985]

If we accept this, there is an apparently insuperable problem. The working-class patient wants help but has only time for a limited number of sessions and is not willing to wait for results; the psycho-analyst wants to help, but insists that the denial of time is the denial of the essence of what she can offer. Psychoanalysis claims the universality of its truth, but sees the *democratization* of its methods as an adulteration. The working-class patient insists on the reality of her social deprivation, the psychoanalyst on the centrality of psychic distortion of reality.

Conclusion

Scarce resources for essential goods and services should be distributed so that basic needs are given priority, irrespective of class, gender, ethnic origin, and other morally irrelevant characteristics. Psychotherapy is, we have argued, such a resource. The expansion and redistribution of psychotherapy which we advocate can be achieved only if psychotherapists are able to overcome a number of serious obstacles. Therapists must be especially sensitive to aspirations—both personal and political—that can be realistically achieved, and in distinguishing between realistic goals and those based on fantasy. Therapy may have a useful role in identifying where fantasy and reality lie. Chasseguet-Smirgel apparently sees only the regressive elements in progressive politics, and she ignores justifiable demands for a more widely available psychotherapy service. At the same time, it is clear that there are important elements of envy-based fantasy in some unrealistic revolutionary objective.

An unequal society is likely to produce an inequitable psychotherapy. To make a simple point: analytic psychotherapy probably requires a certain educational level in patients for it to be effective. A society that has major inequalities in education will therefore be likely to have inequitable psychotherapy. It would certainly be unrealistic and arrogant of psychotherapists to think that they alone could transform society. We have, however, discussed a number of practical measures that would go some way towards redressing the striking imbalance that currently exists in psychotherapy provision. These include the need to increase the total number of psychotherapists at all levels, especially those working in the state-funded service; an emphasis on the importance of "democratic attitudes" among psychotherapists; and the need to modify and broaden psychotherapeutic techniques in order to make them more relevant to a wider range of people.

We can also, at a theoretical level, tentatively suggest an important social role for psychotherapy. It has been suggested by those influenced by the ideas of Melanie Klein—for example, Rustin and Rustin (1984)—that analytic therapy has a particular role in helping with the consequences of deprivation and trauma. On this view, pain and loss may be dealt with in one of two ways: by denial and the emergence of destructive anger that matches the trauma that gave rise to it; or, often with psychotherapeutic help, through the process of grief and mourning that goes beyond anger and depression to a more constructive reparative position. If psychotherapy is to provide this help, the question arises as to whether it is merely palliative, or whether, by facing the reality of socially caused pain and by the working through of loss, grief, and anger to acceptance, it can have a more transformative social role. We shall take up these questions in the next chapter, and again in the final chapter.

CHAPTER FIVE

The social role
of psychotherapy

The previous chapter revealed some of the difficulties of trying to expand psychotherapy in such a way as to make it more accessible to working-class people. One of the major problems seems to be that while conventional psychoanalytic techniques are, for various reasons, unlikely to have widespread popular appeal, the newer therapies are unable, or at least are thought to be unable, to deliver the unique benefits of psychoanalysis. An important reason for this is that one of the central values of psychoanalysis is a commitment to the truth, whereas the newer therapies tend to place a greater emphasis on *change*. We shall discuss the central importance of truth in psychotherapy in subsequent chapters.

This conflict between what we called "high-culture" and popular psychotherapy raises a fundamental moral and political issue about the role that psychotherapy should play within a society, and this forms the focus of the present chapter.

We have been arguing as if it were obvious that more widely available psychotherapy would be desirable were it affordable and arrangeable. The argument is based simply on the claim that what psychotherapy offers its patients by way of emotional autonomy, self-esteem, and the capacity for improved personal relationships is so valuable that people in a relatively affluent society should not be denied its benefits. But this view is controversial even among those who appreciate the effectiveness of psychotherapy. The fear is that too much psychotherapy might, directly or indirectly, be an instrument of social conformity, threatening to suppress individuality and social dissent. It is worth noting that opposition to the expansion of psychotherapy comes not only from right-wing libertarian opponents of the welfare state, whom one would expect to be wary of any expansion of publicly supported welfare services, but also from left-wing social theorists. Rather cheekily, perhaps, we shall call these two groups "the libertarians" and "the Marxists", even though their views are not espoused by all Marxists and libertarians, and are held by some who are neither libertarian nor Marxist.

The Marxist objection

According to Marxism, widespread human misery is inescapable within capitalist society. Apart from brute material poverty, people will be impoverished by living in a world where human relationships are perverted. Neo-Marxists have argued that the inequalities in power, wealth, and dignity which manifest themselves in the workplace are inevitably reproduced within the family.

The pessimistic Freudian account of the human condition maintains that repression of instinctual desire, with its attendant unhappiness, is an inevitable accompaniment of *civilized* society. Marxists have criticized Freud's analysis of the origins of neurosis on the grounds that it mistakes a local truth about capitalist society for a universal biological truth. Many Marxists are, however, prepared to accept the importance of psychoanalysis as an account of the human condition under *capitalism*. These "Freudo–Marxists" believe that the worst conflicts between instinct gratification and civilization are in principle superable. But they can only be conquered if society is transformed.

As we have seen, Freud at one point described his therapeutic work as trying to transform "hysterical misery" into "common unhappiness" (Freud, 1895d). When combined with Freud's pessimistic view about the inevitability of the repression caused by the conflict between civilization and instinct gratification, this idea of the role of therapy looks remarkably like a defence of quietism. Psychoanalysis offers nothing to tackle the underlying causes of unhappiness, which seem to be taken as given; therapy is just a way of helping people to accept their fate, to adjust, and ultimately to settle for quiescent conformity.

This particularly concerns the Freudo–Marxists of the Frankfurt School, of whom Herbert Marcuse is perhaps the best known. They believe that the main obstacle to people working to reduce human misery lies in a failure to understand its true causes—inequalities of power and the *surplus repression* that inescapably accompany capitalism. They are prepared to agree with Freud that any civilization requires some repression of instinct gratification, not least because people have to accommodate each other's needs. They argue, however, that one of the reasons for seeking to replace capitalism with a different kind of society is that it is unable to operate successfully without the stimulation of desires for material possessions, power, and status which at the same time cannot, under capitalism, be satisfied for more than a minority. Under these circumstances, to maintain stability there has to be an extra *repression* of desire, over and above what is needed for civilization as such. They believe that psychoanalytic *theory is* radical in that it reveals how, from earliest childhood, people are oppressed by the inhuman personal relationships which are the product of capitalism. But they are concerned that resort to psychoanalytic *therapy* may help to reinforce social conformity. This fear is clearly expressed by Herbert Marcuse:

> While psychoanalytic theory recognises that the sickness of the individual is ultimately caused and sustained by the sickness of his civilisation, psychoanalytic therapy aims at curing the individual so that he can continue to function as part of a sick civilisation without surrendering to it altogether. [Marcuse, 1966]

The suspicion of Marxists about psychotherapy, particularly about the new, more popular therapies, is that they are in reality subtle devices for making people find the genuinely oppressive and inhuman societies in which they live acceptable, or at least tolerable. This is expressed most strongly by Russell Jacoby (1975). He is particularly critical of "humanistic psychology", of which Carl Rogers is a celebrated exponent:

> Rogers in *Encounter Groups* writes that "the encounter group movement will be a growing counterforce to the dehumanization

of our culture." Proposed is not the dissolution of dehumaniza-
tion, but its humanization. The brutal totality is accepted as
given. . . . One is sensitive toward the immediate and indifferent
toward the more distant social forces which define the immediate. "One of the most imaginative uses [of encounter groups] has
been in dealing with the psychological problems that develop
when two companies merge," writes Rogers. The unholy alliance
between monopoly capital and the Center for Studies of the Person is no sacrilege. The concern of the former for pacifying its
employees, like the concern of the latter, is not malicious but is
grounded in the lie of bourgeois society that they both share: the
ills are subjective. The objective whole is driven from mind by a
program of "feel more, think less." [Jacoby, 1975]

The message seems to be that psychotherapy should be regarded
with great suspicion because, despite the perhaps benign intentions
of its practitioners, it cannot avoid being just a palliative, diverting
attention and energy away from the true causes of human misery: the
inhuman social and political system in which we have to live.

This argument undoubtedly has some force. One of the most repugnant features of life in *Brave New World* is that its inhabitants have
been moulded in such a way that they are almost perfectly adapted to
their environment. They do not even raise questions about the justification of the hierarchical ordering of their society; they just work and
play in an uncritical way. And yet most people would feel that
Bernard Marx, the central character of the novel, who is critical and
consequently dissatisfied, is doing better as a human being than the
masses who are cajoled into calm conformity.

It is also true that psychotherapy, whether for individuals or
for families, is unlikely to eradicate poverty, exploitation, and other
material causes of "common unhappiness". Bettelheim's adolescent
hope (see p. 97)—"that once the vast majority of men had profited
from its [psychoanalysis's] inner liberation they would almost automatically create the good society for themselves"—was just a hope.
To suppose that a good society could be created in this way is grossly
to underestimate the forces that tell against it.

Nevertheless, we should not be carried away by Jacoby's hyperbole. His argument rests on a false dichotomy. In the absence of social
revolution, those who might seek psychotherapy do not face such a
stark choice between an undignified painless conformity and a digni-
fied critical misery. One of the central aims of psychotherapy is to

enable its beneficiaries to become more autonomous, to assume more control over their own lives. Being able to survive psychologically in an unjust, inhuman world is not the same thing as accepting that that world is just, human, or immutable. Here is an example:

THE DEPRESSED DIY SALESMAN

A boy was brought up on a council estate by parents who hoped that he would get on in life and do better than his father, who was an unskilled textile worker. His parents pushed him to do well at school. When he was 16 his father was made redundant, and the family suffered serious financial hardship. The boy felt he had to support his family and left school to get a job in a new do-it-yourself superstore. Shortly after this, he started having rows with his parents about his staying out late and not fulfilling their hopes "after all we have done for you". He became very depressed, went to his doctor, and was referred to a psychotherapist. After an assessment interview, the therapist told him that he would like to see him with his parents. Family therapy helped him to feel less responsible for the welfare of the whole family, and helped his parents to allow him more freedom. After ten sessions he had regained his joie de vivre and returned to work, where in time he became a successful store manager.

From the bare details given here, one could interpret this as confirming Jacoby's fear. The real causes of the boy's depression were not that there was something pathological about him, or about his family. Rather, they lay in the fact that his circumstances prevented him from doing what he and his parents really wanted. He was put in an impossible position, where no matter what he did would be unsatisfactory. The solution to his problems, and to those of thousands like him, it might be argued, is not to give them therapy but to change the social and political structures that lead to this kind of dilemma.

This line of thought does not, however, constitute a criticism of *psychotherapy* without the addition of highly dubious premises. Let us grant that the boy's material circumstances *did* cause his depression. It does not follow that nothing should be done short of changing the circumstances. Such a conclusion rests on two possible misconceptions.

The first is about causality. It is misleading to speak as if there were *one* cause of something as complex as a person's depression.

Any event has an indefinite number of causally relevant factors, each of which is necessary and together are jointly sufficient for the occurrence of the event. When we loosely speak of *the* cause, we are referring to that factor among all the causally relevant factors upon which, for our own purposes, we wish to focus—usually to apportion moral or legal blame.

In our example, it may well be true that the material circumstances of the boy and his family were necessary conditions of his becoming depressed. It may also be true that, unless there is a change in the organization of society, he and thousands of others like him will be especially prone to depression. However, this is consistent with the possibility that another causally necessary factor in his becoming and remaining depressed was his failure to realize that his situation was placing impossible psychological demands upon him— to satisfy his parents' contradictory desires that he should support them financially and yet simultaneously continue his formal education. Therapy helped him to realize that he should not blame himself for failing to live up to his parents' idealized and impossible views about what he should do.

The second misconception is that enabling people to tolerate or cope with adverse circumstances is tantamount to cajoling them into conformist acceptance of those circumstances. It might be that, given the real, material constraints placed on him by society, the best option for the boy in our example *was* to work vigorously in the superstore. He could do this without believing that such a solution was ideal, and still maintain an open mind for possibilities of breaking out when the time was right. Jacoby is too pessimistic in his rejection of the worth of psychotherapeutic intervention in an inhuman world when he writes:

> The fetish of human relations, responses, emotions, perpetuates the myth; abstracted from the social whole they appear as the individualized responses of free men and women to particular situations and not, as they are, the subhuman responses to a nonhuman world. ... The endless talk of human relations and responses is utopian; it assumes what is obsolete or yet to be realized: *human* relations. Today these relations are inhuman; they partake more of rats than of humans, more of things than of people. And not because of bad will but because of an evil society. To forget this is to indulge in the ideology of sensitivity groups that work to desensitize by cutting off human relations

from the social roots that have made them brutal. More sensitivity today means revolution or madness. The rest is chatter.
[Jacoby, 1975]

Suppose it *is* true that the society we live in is oppressive, and that
unless the fundamental power relations in society are transformed
many people will continue to suffer from anxiety, alienation, depression, and overall unhappiness. It *would* follow that even *widespread*
psychotherapy could not on its own provide a lasting and universal
solution to the problems with which it deals, but *not* that psychotherapy is an obstacle to progressive social change, keeping people
quiet and diverting attention away from the gross injustices that per-
vade the world in which we live.

Indeed, following our arguments of the previous two chapters,
we would argue that, compared with other approaches to the treatment of psychological distress, psychotherapy is the least likely to
produce social conformity, since one of its main vehicles for change is
helping patients to understand their situation better. To advocate an
expansion of the availability of psychotherapy, as we do, is entirely
consistent with recognizing that much misery is socially caused, and
that *social* change as well as psychotherapy is, in the long run, essential for reducing that misery.

Psychotherapy is not an alternative to social and political activ-
ism. Although it cannot by itself eliminate the social, political, and
economic causes of human misery, there is no reason why it could not
be used as a weapon against these by those seeking to transform
society for the better. Emotional autonomy is likely to make people
more effective and less malleable, rather than quietist. The one significant area of psychotherapy which *might* seriously lend itself to the
abuse of trying to impose social conformity is behaviour therapy,
especially when it is used in contexts of coercion. In chapter eight, we
discuss the specific problems raised by this, which is rather a special
case.

The libertarian objection

If psychotherapy were to be regarded as a part of essential care that
should be available to people according to need, then, like medical
care and education, it would require substantial public funding, since

not everyone who needs psychotherapy can afford it. We have tried in previous chapters to rebut the pragmatic objection to state-funded psychotherapy: that it would be a waste of resources. We shall now consider a *principled* objection to such a development, which comes from the libertarian radical right.

Perhaps the most famous opponent of institutional state-organized psychiatry and, by extension, psychotherapy is the American psychoanalyst Thomas Szasz. In his book *The Manufacture of Madness*, Szasz (1973) argues that the psychiatric profession and the institutions of psychiatry have been used, wittingly or unwittingly, as mechanisms for enforcing certain moral standards. He compares psychiatry to the Spanish Inquisition, and the treatment of mental patients to the persecution of witches and heretics.

He cites numerous historical examples of psychiatry, backed up by the coercive powers of the state, being used to persecute "deviants": masturbators, homosexuals, unmarried mothers, and cannabis smokers, among others. In the following passage he describes a dilemma that he thinks confronts all psychiatrists who are employed by a public authority:

> The physician who decides to be an institutional psychiatrist puts himself, though he may do so unwittingly, into [the following] predicament: he must choose between roasting—that is, being an agent of the state, stigmatizing innocent individuals as malefactors; and being roasted—that is, being an agent of the persecuted mental patient, risking being branded by his colleagues, as deviant, uncooperative, irresponsible as a physician, or even mad himself. On the other hand, the psychiatrist who decides to work as a private psychotherapist, as for example, some psychoanalysts may do, may transcend this dilemma, by choosing, with Abraham Lincoln, the dimension of equality and non-coercion. "As I would not be a slave, so I would not be a master," said Lincoln. "This expresses my idea of democracy. Whatever differs from this, to the extent of the difference is not democracy." [Szasz, 1973]

Szasz's argument from the history of psychiatry has considerable polemical appeal, but it is greatly weakened by his reliance on highly selective evidence. He takes the worst abuses of compulsory detention and treatment of mental patients, and represents these abuses as typical. There is no argument over whether or not state-institutionalized psychiatry has been used to oppress *some* patients, and to suppress *some* patients' freedom to express their individuality. It has. But this can be accepted by those who advocate the development of state-supported psychotherapy. The crucial questions for the present argument are: "Would state-funded psychotherapy inevitably persecute 'innocent individuals'?" and "Are the alternatives to state funding better or worse?"

We do not think that Szasz's main argument from the history of psychiatry ought to persuade anyone that state-funded psychotherapy is a dangerous instrument of social control by sinister agents of state power. There are two reasons for this. First, his claims about psychiatry are exaggerated; second, even if true of *psychiatry*, they cannot plausibly be extended to *psychotherapy*.

We believe that Szasz's claim about the plight of psychiatrists working in state institutions rests on a false dichotomy. It is an absurd exaggeration to say that any psychiatrist who is an employee of the state faces a stark choice between "stigmatizing innocent individuals as malefactors" and genuinely helping their patients only at the risk of "being branded by his colleagues as deviant, uncooperative, irresponsible as a physician, or even mad himself".

The image conjured up is of the state psychiatrist wandering round his hospital administering powerful tranquillizing drugs and electric shocks to victimized, incarcerated patients whose only crime is to deviate from prevailing cultural norms. This is highly misleading, especially in the light of the fact that the numbers of compulsory detainees in state mental institutions have declined rapidly over the past two decades.

Of course, given the subject-matter of psychiatry, it is always possible for governments to abuse it in such a way as to punish various types of non-conformity, and to stifle the fundamental freedom of dissent. However, whether or not there is such abuse will depend on the political style and power of the government, rather than on whether or not psychiatry is publicly funded. A state may use its institutions for worse *or* better purposes. In this respect, state-funded psychotherapy is no exception.

This brings us to our second major reason for resisting Szasz's challenge to state-funded psychotherapy. Even if it were true of state-financed institutional *psychiatry* that it has been used in a deplorable way as an instrument of enforcing conformity, this is much less likely to be true of the kind of *psychotherapy* service that we are proposing.

Psychiatric patients in hospital who receive formal psychotherapy —and there are scandalously few—are very rarely compulsorily detained. Nearly all state-funded psychotherapy patients attend hospital out-patients' departments or day hospitals voluntarily. Furthermore, there is no reason to equate state-funded psychotherapy, or even modern state-funded psychiatry, with the large institutions that have traditionally housed the insane.

In fact, opposition to the worst aspects of institutional psychiatry usually goes hand-in-hand with a commitment to psychotherapy. Many of the small community mental health centres that are replacing the large mental hospitals are run along psychotherapeutic lines. In contrast to Szasz's analysis, most defenders of publicly funded psychotherapy are also well aware of the dangers of psychiatric abuse, and are among its strongest critics. Sidney Bloch, a staunch advocate of state-funded psychotherapy, was at the forefront of a campaign to end psychiatric abuse in the Soviet Union before soviet communism collapsed. He graphically described the plight of a small group of pre-*perestroika* Soviet dissenters who

> have been diagnosed, although mentally well, as suffering from such serious psychiatric conditions as schizophrenia and paranoid personality disorder. As a result of their "illness", they have been detained involuntarily in ordinary or prison psychiatric hospitals for periods ranging from weeks to many years. While in hospital some have been given tranquillising and other drugs for which they have no need; the purpose rather has been to use medication as form of social control. All have experienced the severe trauma of being placed alongside genuinely ill patients; the fear of not knowing when, and indeed whether, they would be released; and some the indignity of being pressed to recant their dissenting views, often held with considerable conviction and over many years, in order to signify their "recovery" and expedite their release. [Bloch, 1981]

Szasz's nightmarish scenario of a state-funded psychotherapy service being used to attempt to brainwash or demoralize dissidents is far from the realities of a liberal democracy. In any case, if a state's authorities *were* intent on using the treatment of the mentally ill as a form of social control, the drugs used by doctors and psychiatrists would be a cheaper and more effective weapon. Nevertheless, it is important that there should be some way of ensuring that therapists, whether private or publicly funded, do not abuse their power. We discuss this further in chapters eight and nine.

Even if it *were* true that there is some risk of psychotherapy being abused by the state as a way of promoting conformity, it certainly would not follow, as Szasz would have us think, that psychotherapy should be restricted to those who are able to enter into a financial contract for treatment with a private therapist.

The main force of the anti–state-power argument seems to rest on the assumption that all institutions of the state inevitably restrict individual freedom. This is trivially true, if we equate individual freedom with that area of a person's life which lies outside the concern of the state. But the assumption is hard to sustain if we think of freedom more substantively, as autonomy or the capacity to control one's own life. It is admittedly true that paternalistic restrictions on people's choices often stunt or suppress their autonomy. It is also true that public funding of any activity restricts the liberty of those who are compelled to contribute to the public funding through taxation. But we are not advocating the development of paternalistic, compulsory psychotherapy; and against the loss of freedom for those who would have to contribute towards the funding of an expanded psychotherapy service, there has to be balanced the enormous gains in autonomy that therapy offers its beneficiaries. One of the main contentions is that a distinctive aim of psychotherapy is the promotion of personal emotional autonomy. The psychotherapies that we have been defending aim to enable their beneficiaries to become more autonomous, to be less dominated by wayward emotions, to gain a better understanding of their situations, and to be able to face up to painful facts about their own lives. These are all ways of enhancing freedom.

This leads directly to a third reason for rejecting Szasz's conclusion. If psychotherapy were available, as Szasz would like, simply for those able "freely" to negotiate a contract with a private therapist (that is, for an unsubsidized fee), many who needed it would be denied the opportunity to have psychotherapy. It is one thing to argue, in the name of freedom, that nobody should be *forced* to have psychotherapy or any other sort of treatment for the mind. It is quite another to argue, in the name of freedom, that there should be provision only for those who can pay. This would be a plausible view only if people's need for psychotherapy were directly related to their disposable income—an absurd hypothesis, albeit one that Szasz, on occasion, seems to espouse. His dismissive view of the chances of emotional autonomy for the less well-off is captured in the following quotation from his book *The Ethics of Psychoanalysis*. He is here writing specifically about psychoanalysis, which we see as only one kind of essential psychotherapeutic care. But he would, presumably, say the same things about other forms of psychotherapy, which we would also wish to see made much more widely available.

> The poor need jobs and money, not psychoanalysis. The uneducated need knowledge and skills, not psychoanalysis. Furthermore, the poor and the uneducated are also often politically disfranchised and socially oppressed; if this is the case, they need freedom from oppression. The kind of *personal* freedom that psychoanalysis promises can have meaning only for persons who enjoy a large measure of economic, political and social freedom. [Szasz, 1969]

It is no doubt true that psychotherapy is not the most pressing need for people who are literally starving. But Szasz's argument, like the Marxist's, rests on a false dichotomy—between jobs and money on the one hand, and psychotherapy on the other. Of course we accept that "the poor" need jobs, money, and freedom from oppression; but some of them need psychotherapy as well, and we do not accept that the provision of the one excludes provision of the other. Even though psychoanalysis may be unsuitable for inarticulate, less well-educated people, the same is not true for all psychotherapies. And there is certainly no plausible psychological theory according to which neurosis, anxiety, and depression, and the possibility of transcending them, arise only with wealth, employment, and education.

It is both interesting and disturbing how an unholy alliance between Marxists and the New Right can serve to undermine the chances of psychotherapy becoming more widely available to those who need it. In trying to set out a positive social role for psychotherapy, it is useful to consider analogies between psychotherapy and two other controversial social institutions—Third World aid and education. The analogies are instructive in bringing out the dynamic of the middle ground being attacked by both left- and right-wing dogmatism.

Aid, first aid, and fundamental change

There is a popular, though flawed, argument, used by people of various political persuasions, against expanding, or even maintaining, food aid to the Third World. According to the left-wing version of the argument, we should not give such aid because by providing aid we are prolonging the viability of corrupt, unjust regimes, thus delaying the radical social change that would tackle the problem at source. It is vital, in particular, to change the land tenure system in many parts of the world, which guarantees that, no matter how much overseas aid is provided, millions will remain at or near starvation levels. Aid is at best diversionary, and at worst actively harms those it is meant to benefit, by keeping them in a state of permanent dependency.

A right-wing version, exemplified by Garrett Hardin (1979), claims that people need to be taught the hard way to stand on their own feet. Hardin believes that continued aid will weaken incentives both for poor and rich in Third World countries to act in a socially responsible way. The poor will have no reason to become responsible for their own lives if someone else will pick up the pieces; and the rich will lose the incentive for good housekeeping if its benefits are to be distributed apparently without limit to the ever-increasing poor. Providing aid is thus allegedly bad for providers and recipients alike. Of particular interest in this context is the claim that aid is harmful to its recipients since, whether or not by design, it fosters long-term helplessness and dependency of the malign sort.

Similar arguments have been produced against social and community work. According to the left-wing version, these caring professions are inevitably reactionary, since their chief function, irrespective of the intentions of individual social and community workers, is to enable the basically unjust and inhuman society—which creates the need for these professions—to continue. The right-wing version appeals to the value of self-reliance. People will never be self-reliant, and therefore free, unless they have the opportunity to take responsibility for their own lives. The "nanny state" is to be deplored since it undermines the incentive for the less fortunate members of society to take care of themselves properly. This is bad for them, and bad for the more able and better off who will be held back by the burden of having to support the large demands of the less fortunate.

These are reminiscent of arguments brought against psychotherapy. On the one hand, it is argued that psychotherapy, with its concentration on individual liberation, is diversionary and obstructs necessary fundamental social change. On the other, it is argued that entrusting one's emotional life to state-supported experts prevents individuals from properly standing on their own feet. Maybe life is difficult, but it undermines human freedom if it becomes normal for people always to look to others, particularly to the state, to sort out their emotional difficulties.

Both these arguments have a rhetorical appeal derived from the grain of truth that each contains. When examined dispassionately, however, they collapse.

Anyone who thinks that the problems of Third World poverty and famine could be solved by food aid is at best extremely naive. But although this is true, as are analogous observations about social work and psychotherapy, it does not justify the conclusion that aid should be stopped, restricted, or not expanded. If there were a simple choice between offering food aid now or successfully reforming the land tenure system, educating everyone about birth control, and eliminating water-borne diseases, a strong case could be made for restricting food aid. But there is no reason why food aid should exclude the other measures. The incentives and ability to control family size and to become more self-reliant come with economic and social development. In so far as the aid does not prevent such development, it need not generate permanent dependency. Indeed, aid may, in the short term, be a prerequisite for independence.

As far as radical social change is concerned, historical evidence suggests that starvation is likely to be an obstacle rather than a facilitator. On the other hand, there is no reason in principle why aid programmes should not be targeted differently so that they help those who need them most, or help those who will benefit most, and designed in such a way as to promote the long-term independence of the beneficiaries of the aid. The fact that many existing aid programmes do not work well is not an argument against aid in general, but only against current forms of aid. It would turn into a comprehensive argument against aid only if it could be shown that it is impossible for aid to take the benign form suggested here. We do not believe that this could be shown.

What about psychotherapy? We have already discussed the fears that state-funded psychotherapy may be just a palliative, sustaining a corrupt and unjust society, and a way of taking individual responsibility and freedom away from people.

The reply to both sets of criticisms concedes the truth in each. Psychotherapy alone will not transform society, and it *is* desirable that people should take responsibility for their own lives. But these concessions do not undermine the main case for psychotherapy. Those who are concerned about the creation of a society where citizens are lulled into conformity by a welfare state concerned with mental health should turn their attention elsewhere—to *tranquillizers*, for example—rather than psychotherapy.

It is almost indisputable that tranquillizers have been overprescribed by beleaguered doctors who do not have the time to offer psychotherapeutic help which might elucidate the problems that have led their patients to be anxious, depressed, neurotic, or alienated. One result of this is that millions of people throughout the world have become addicted to benzodiazepines such as Ativan and Valium. These drugs are often prescribed over long periods, even though they are safe and effective only in the short term. The use of tranquillizers by doctors, wittingly or unwittingly, *does* seem to illustrate how attention may be diverted away from fundamental problems. A tranquillizer can never be more than a palliative that just enables people to carry on—somehow—without trying to come to terms with the real problems of their lives. The risks of benzodiazepine over-prescription are graphically, if somewhat sensationally, described in Vernon Coleman's *Life Without Tranquillisers*:

> Quite apart from the risks to individual consumers of these tablets, capsules and medicines there is, I believe, an enormous risk to our society. Individuals who take benzodiazepines become numbed and easily moulded, they tend to accept things without protest, and they feel little in the way of emotional responses. That's the way benzodiazepines work—they turn anxious, worried human beings into zombies. Giving up the drugs is difficult because it means being exposed to a whole range of frightening and disturbing stimuli. The benzodiazepine user gets hooked because life *with* Valium is comfortable and undemanding. [Coleman, 1985]

To return to the analogy with the Third World: the use of tranquillizers is like the provision of grain hand-outs. Or to use another analogy, it is like first aid. In a crisis like that which faced Ethiopia and the Sudan in 1985, where people are actually starving to death and there is an abundance of grain elsewhere that could be used to feed them, it would be monstrous to withhold the grain. To do so would be to place virtually no weight on the interests of the starving. However, the underlying problems that cause starvation will certainly not be *solved* by grain hand-outs. Those seeking to address these problems must turn their attention to international "agribusiness" and the inequalities of power within Third World countries (George, 1979). But there is no inconsistency between this and giving aid to organizations and even individuals in poor countries. The aid should, however, be directed, as far as possible, towards increasing the independence of the victims of poverty, so that ultimately they are able to take effective steps to overcome it, even if this requires radical economic and social changes.

Tranquillizers can occasionally be helpful in overcoming the immediate effects of acute anxiety and insomnia that can result from sudden shock or trauma like bereavement or divorce. The immediate beneficial effects last for about ten to fourteen days, after which the tranquillizers become less effective. Long-term use of tranquillizers almost invariably prevents patients from assuming more responsibility for their own lives; they are addictive and may divert their users from facing up to the problems that generated the anxiety or depression in the first place. It is true that psychotherapy alone cannot eradicate the material causes of these problems. But, compared with tranquillizers, it can hardly be claimed that therapy is either diversionary or likely to generate long-term dependency.

There are many different ways of surviving emotional stress. Among the least attractive is to become dependent on tranquillizers or other autonomy-reducing drugs. Tranquillizers offer a "solution" that is really an admission of defeat—an admission that the patient is not to be entrusted with facing the *reality* of her own life. Even if psychotherapy were, like drug therapies, primarily symptom-directed, it would have a value. But it is not: it offers much more. Psychotherapy does not provide an escape from reality, but positively encourages its users to confront the reasons why they are miserable: it aims directly at enhancing autonomy.

The role that we would like to see for psychotherapy is analogous to the progressive forms of aid mentioned above. The fact that psychotherapy cannot transform society and eradicate the social causes of mental distress is no argument against its usefulness in helping the casualties of civilization or, if one accepts the Freudo–Marxist view, of capitalist repression. People who, through psychotherapy, become less crippled by anxiety, depression, or neurosis may become more effective in the pursuit of whatever goals they have, including the goal of working for the transformation of society.

Education and psychotherapy

In the previous chapter, we introduced an analogy between psychotherapy and education, in the context of "high" and popular culture. There we concentrated on the educational needs of adults—arguing that life in an Oxford research college, although of unique value, is unlikely to be an appropriate medium for making further and higher education available to all who need it. We develop the educational analogy further here, but this time in another direction.

In the years before the Industrial Revolution, formal education was almost exclusively the preserve of the middle and upper classes. From an "enlightened" twentieth-century perspective, this seems to have constituted a significant aspect of the ways in which the poor were oppressed. All children have a right to education, and a civilized society should ensure that they all receive it.

Ignorance is not itself a form of illness or deviancy, but an inevitable accompaniment of youth and inexperience. Formal education for children is necessary because in a complex, competitive world it may be impossible for them to function effectively without it. Ideally, education offers children a way of learning to read, write, become numerate, acquire a general understanding of the world that they live in, and become autonomous, yet good, citizens. Education, although offering something of great benefit, is not, like the treatment of disease, an attempt to stamp out something pathological. Childhood and ignorance are not diseases. Of course people may have varying educational needs and capabilities, and some, with "special educational needs", may have deficiencies that *are* pathological. They need special care within the education system.

If we accept that anxiety, depression, and neurosis are, in varying degrees, an inevitable accompaniment of life in a complex modern society, it is not absurd to maintain that psychotherapy should have a role similar to education. Probably most people could benefit from psychotherapy at some point in their lives. As things stand, at least 10 per cent of the population have *psychiatric* treatment at some stage. The fact that people *do* need therapy, in the sense that therapy could make them less unhappy, neurotic, or anxious, does not mean that they are sick. Periods of anxiety and depression are no less a normal condition for adults at certain times in their lives—for example, following a bereavement—than is ignorance for a child. Therapy offers people the chance of understanding their own psychological distress, and of overcoming it in autonomy-enhancing ways. Of course, some people *do* have special psychological needs, just as some children have special educational needs, and ideally they would receive more intensive or prolonged psychotherapeutic care.

In the lively debate preceding the passing of the 1870 Education Act, which recognized for the first time in England that education should be a public service, great hope was expressed that education could transform society. The social role of education would be to enable people, particularly the working class, to develop their higher human intellectual capacities to the full. The hope was that this would lead to a more harmonious society of citizens who would, in pursuit of their own individuality, serve the interests of the whole community. This is given clear expression in John Stuart Mill's discussion of happiness, which we considered in chapter three.

Let us recall that, for Mill, happiness consists of a life which is relatively pain-free and relatively pleasant, with great variety, a decided predominance of active over passive pleasures, and a realistic understanding of what life can offer—both its possibilities and its limitations:

> A life thus composed, to those who have been fortunate enough to obtain it, has always appeared worthy of the name of happiness. And such an existence is even now the lot of many, during some considerable portion of their lives. *The present wretched education, and wretched social arrangements* are the only real hindrance to its being attainable by almost all. [Mill, 1861; italics added]

Mill, the great liberal, whom Szasz quotes as a champion of the individual against the state, believed that education should be available to all children. Indeed, Mill believed that education should be compulsory. The reasons for making education compulsory for children up to a certain age have to do with the special vulnerabilities of children, and the fear that many parents would not allow their children to go to school unless they were made to. Mill believed that all children should have the benefit of education. He regarded it as a proper duty of society to ensure that no child was denied education through the inability of parents to pay. The state should, therefore, subsidize education. He was at pains to point out, however, the difference between the state paying for education and the state's attempting to control the specific content of education, which he opposed.

Although in recent years governments have taken an increasingly active role in trying to define the curriculum in schools, there is no reason why state funding of education should necessitate central state control of its content. Indeed, there is a good case for arguing that at least the detailed content of even state-funded education should be negotiated by parents, teachers, and, where appropriate, pupils.

We have argued that there is a good case for making psychotherapy available to all who need it, irrespective of ability to pay. Like universal education, this would require substantial public funding, although for obvious reasons, unlike education, it would not require compulsion. By analogy with education, it is important to distinguish the state's funding of psychotherapy from state control of the details of its practice.

In view of the arguments put forward in chapter four about the appropriateness of different types of therapy for different people, we would strongly advocate that there should be a diversity of therapies available, and that the content and direction of therapy should not be closely controlled by a centralized state authority. On the other hand, there is a need to ensure that proper standards are maintained. We argue in later chapters that the best vehicle to achieve this goal would be an independent professional council of psychotherapy and the introduction of a register of psychotherapists.

It might seem absurd, in this age of cut-backs and ever-increasing demands on public expenditure, to be even suggesting something like publicly funded psychotherapy for all who need it. It may well be, however, that we are blinkered by the fact that we have so far got by without it, in just the way that the early Victorians were blinkered about education.

In spite of the optimism of the pro-educationists such as Mill, there was stubborn resistance to the expansion of education. Apart from the sheer cost, it was feared that education would give the poor ideas "above their station". Universal education was opposed primarily on three grounds: that it would actually be harmful to the working class in that it would raise their expectations; that this would lead to social instability; and that it was in any case a waste of time and money.

Yet there was a certain inevitability about the development of education. It was economically necessary in a developing industrial society to have a literate work force. School was an ideal place for teaching children respect for authority and about working closely with large numbers of other people. These may have been a far cry from what Mill envisaged, but they were all important factors in the development of education. According to the historian James Walvin,

> much of the value of a national education lay outside its ability to educate. Education was important in removing from the streets and alleyways those children who had so plagued society and taxed the popular imagination. Many Victorian writers had been exercised with the problems of what to do with these children. . . . To have all the nation's children in the classrooms during much of the working day, throughout a substantial part of the year, fulfilled a number of important social roles. After a fashion it brought the children under control, it expanded employment opportunities, particularly for young women, and permitted parents and relatives to escape from the tedious tasks of child-minding to take up paid employment. [Walvin, 1982]

When progressive reforms such as the decision to provide education for all are implemented, it is not usually the moral arguments alone that win the day. Rather, there are always sound reasons of political and economic expediency which operate on those in power in such a way as to make the moral arguments suddenly sound persuasive. In spite of this, education always has the potential for enabling students to become more critical of existing power relations, less easy to keep in subservience, more autonomous. These are by-products of even conformist education.

What about psychotherapy? It could be argued that late twentieth-century Western society is facing an internal crisis, which has generated a need for psychotherapy that is stronger than ever. The family is threatened by an ever-increasing incidence of divorce; traditional attitudes towards work are being threatened by record long-term unemployment; labour mobility is destroying the stability of local communities; and religion has declined. Some of these changes may even be beneficial in the long run, but each greatly increases levels of anxiety, depression, neurosis, and alienation. Together, they threaten the cohesion of society, perhaps to just as great an extent as the roaming children threatened the stability of Victorian Britain.

Psychotherapy may, like education in the nineteenth century, become socially necessary, as social cohesion diminishes and psychological distress increases. Education is, irrespective of the designs of educators, inherently subversive. So, too—because of its emphasis on facing personal and social reality, and its search for change, however modest, rather than conformity—is psychotherapy.

In such a climate there is, in spite of recent attempts to reduce public spending, a great opportunity for the dramatic extension of psychotherapeutic services. Although, as we have argued, the moral case for such an extension is strong, history shows that in the end it is likely to be economic and political expediency that determine broad policy. We believe that this *will* lead eventually to a large expansion of psychotherapy services. It is especially important that policy-makers, practitioners, and the public are kept aware of the moral arguments, and that in the implementation of policies there are proper safeguards to prevent the abuse of psychotherapy and to protect the rights of users and practitioners.

CHAPTER SIX

The therapeutic relationship: ethical implications of transference

Practitioners would, on the whole, rather think about technique than ethics. The embryologist studying the newly fertilized ovum is more concerned with working out how differentiation of the nervous system occurs than with the ethical issue of when an embryo acquires rights. Ethical issues lie at the *boundaries* of everyday practice, and clinicians, like football players, want to get on with the game rather than argue endlessly about rules and infringements. Passions may become momentarily inflamed, which is why referees are needed, but the less they have to intervene the better the game.

From this perspective, medical ethics—and, by extension, psychotherapeutic ethics—could be seen as concerned with questions to which no *technical* solution can be found within medicine or psychotherapy itself. Biochemistry alone will never indicate when to switch off a ventilator for a patient in a coma, or whether a managing director is more deserving of renal dialysis than a tramp.

Science and physical medicine have an advantage over psychotherapy in that at least in them the distinction between technique and ethics is usually fairly clear. In psychotherapy, the position is more complicated: the very subject-matter is a focus of moral dispute, and the moral choices faced by patients are the bread and butter of psychotherapy sessions. Should a therapist help an unhappy couple to stay together, or encourage an oppressed and intimidated wife to leave? How can therapists persuade suicidal patients that life is worth living? How far should therapists go in offering lonely patients friendship and support? Should a patient who is low in self-esteem be told that she is attractive and intelligent, or would this be seductive and perhaps lead to unproductive dependency on the therapist—and if she is not, would it not be dishonest to say she is? Is it justifiable to tell "white lies" to patients if it will help them to get better: should the therapist reassure patients that they *will* improve (as Freud is said to have done at times) in spite of being secretly doubtful about the outcome? Should the therapist reveal something of her own difficulties, in the hope that this will make the patient feel less isolated?

Given the subject-matter of psychotherapy, it is often tempting for therapists to become active participants in the patient's life and therefore, where necessary, to give advice, be self-revealing, and generally become the patient's moral accomplice and mentor. From this perspective, ethics might seem all-important on the grounds that, since the whole field of psychotherapy is value-laden, no clear demarcation between technique and ethics, between play and boundaries, can be drawn, and so, to paraphrase Marshall McLuhan, the message (or interpretation) is the morality.

In this chapter, we adopt a different viewpoint. We strongly believe that technique is as important in psychotherapy as in any other profession. We show how, through the use of technical psychoanalytic concepts of transference and countertransference, some of the apparent ethical dilemmas of everyday psychotherapy practice can be resolved within the boundaries of technique. By taking transference and countertransference into account, the touchline of psychotherapy remains in place, allowing play to proceed uninterrupted. Ultimately, of course, ethical boundaries *are* reached. It is as mistaken to argue that ethical questions can, through correct technique, be avoided altogether, as it is to confuse what is basically a transferential issue with one of ethics.

The popular view of transference might be that it is "falling in love with your analyst". Contemporary psychoanalysis takes a wider view than this, recognizing that there are unconscious aspects that operate continuously in any interaction between therapist and patient. Transference refers to the ways in which the feelings, wishes, and actions of the patient in relation to the therapist may be unconsciously influenced, coloured, and distorted by earlier childhood experiences, especially those with parents. Countertransference, on the other hand, comprises both the therapist's "blind-spots"—her unconscious and childhood-derived wishes and fantasies in relation to the patient—and affective responses of which she is aware, which can be put to good use in helping her to understand the patient.

Transference can arise in two contexts. In "everyday" or fleeting transference, prior hopes, fears, expectations, assumptions, and fantasies impinge on interactions with doctors, therapists, and other helpers but are not necessarily encouraged or focused on. "Deep" transference is an extension and exaggeration of everyday transference occurring mainly, but not exclusively, in analytic therapies whose arrangements—for example, the passivity and reticence of the analyst—are especially designed to evoke it.

The moral issues raised by non-analytic therapies are considered in more detail in subsequent chapters. Non-analytic therapists might argue that they have no particular need to consider the ethical implications of transference. We believe, however, that because therapists are inevitably important figures in their patients' lives, and because emotional arousal is a central issue in most therapies, "everyday" transference is likely to be an ingredient in them, whether recognized or not. When difficulties arise in therapy, it is often because transference and countertransference are not being acknowledged. If this is so, it is important for non-analytic therapists to ensure that they are aware of transference and countertransference and their ethical implications, even though, or perhaps just because, it is not central to their thinking and practice.

THE "CRADLE SNATCHER" AND HER HUSBAND

A depressed patient under the care of a female psychiatrist did well in hospital, but he relapsed and became suicidal whenever he went home for the weekend. His wife was very upset by this and demanded a "second opinion" for her husband. He had tried to hang himself the previous weekend, but this, the wife felt, was not being taken seriously; she had been told by the psychiatrist that her husband was "like a child" and must be treated accordingly. This was her second marriage, his first; she was ten years older than him; they had one child of their own, and she had a grown-up daughter by her first marriage who had recently had a baby.

When she saw the second consultant, a psychotherapist, she reiterated that she had been told it was her husband's right to change doctors. It was clear, however, that he, the patient, was quite satisfied with the consultant in whose care he was. It then emerged that he resented his wife's preoccupation with her new grandchild, while she had always felt that he cared more about his mother (from whom she had been accused of "cradle-snatching" him at the age of 19) than about her. This resentment of her mother-in-law in turn linked with her feelings towards her own mother, whom she saw as domineering and idealizing her brother who had died in an accident at the age of 10. He, on the other hand, had clung to his mother throughout childhood and had resented the drunken intrusions of his father, who had been away in the Services for many years. It was clear that this whole pattern had transferred itself on to the first consultant, who, for the wife, had taken on the part of the mother-in-law/mother who ignored her feelings, while for the patient she had become the over-protective mother. Once this was unravelled, the need for a change of doctors disappeared; the original consultant continued to treat them, and they went away for an enjoyable weekend alone, safe from the demands and restrictions of step-grandchildren and mothers-in-law.

Models of the therapist

Before we can tease out the technical and ethical components of the therapeutic relationship and the moral responsibilities of therapists, we must first decide what sort of relationship it is. Psychotherapists have been likened to traders, priests, advocates, pedagogues, parents, and doctors. No doubt there is some truth in all these comparisons, but we find each of them in important ways wanting, and we shall argue that there are some special features of psychotherapy, especially the use of transference and countertransference, that make it and its moral responsibilities unique.

The psychotherapist as trader

We have already discussed the opposition of the psychoanalyst Thomas Szasz to paternalism within the helping professions (Szasz, 1974). As far as he is concerned, the psychotherapist is a trader: the analyst sells something and the patient buys it. If the patient does not like what she is offered, she can go elsewhere. Therapists do not need to worry too much about ethics: the market-place will do that for them. If they are no good, then their patients will go away, and the therapists will lose business. If they are good they will succeed, and such success is sufficient to define their goodness. The problem with this appealingly simple approach is that it fails to take account of some central features of the psychotherapeutic relationship.

The patient is usually not in the position of a free purchaser. She is in distress and is prone to grasp uncritically at any offer of help. The market does not protect old ladies whose pipes burst in winter from exorbitant and incompetent plumbers, and, *a fortiori*, the desperation of someone in need of therapy may frequently lead to bad therapy choices being made by patients.

Psychotherapy is similar to plumbing or legal advice in that each offers a service. However, the psychotherapist is not offering a purely technical service which the patient receives, but a *relationship* in which the patient is as much an active participant as the therapist.

Szasz is unusual in being simultaneously opposed to "welfarism" and a supporter of psychoanalysis. But his gadfly critique of indiscriminate care in psychotherapy does contain an important truth about the psychotherapeutic relationship: in psychotherapy, just as in a commercial transaction, there must be responsibility and willingness on both sides. For psychotherapy to work, the patient must actively *want* it, rather than just passively accept it, and be prepared to give something up in order to achieve success in therapy. Unlike Szasz, however, we do not think that the patient's commitment must necessarily be financial. She may give up time, mistrust, or the known certainty of her neurosis. Because markets are likely to exclude or exploit the poor and the weak, Szasz's approach creates problems just as great, if different from, those associated with the welfare state to which he is so opposed.

For these reasons, we reject Szasz's model of the therapeutic relationship and with it many of his practical recommendations.

The psychotherapist as priest

For Szasz, a therapist's *personal* values are unimportant. What matters is freedom of contract. A very different view has been put forward by authors like Philip Rieff (1979) and Paul Halmos (1965). They see the psychotherapist's own value system as central to the therapeutic relationship. Rieff sees psychotherapy as a form of "moral pedagogy", and therapists as latter-day priests who wrap up their covert moral message in a pseudo-scientific garb.

In his view, it is only a short step from the confessional to the couch: "Psychoanalysis creates little communions of counter-belief ... therapeutic communities of two" (Rieff, 1979). He characterizes Freud's "fundamental rule" of psychoanalysis—the "candour" expected of the patient—as a sacrament, an equivalent to monastic vows of poverty, chastity, and obedience.

For Rieff, psychoanalytic jargon represents an attempt to disguise moral discourse as science:

> What is for Freud "repression" psychologically understood, is "secrecy" morally understood. Secrecy is [a] category of moral illness, for it provides a hiding place for false motives. It is our secrets, hidden from ourselves, that fester and infect action. [Rieff, 1979]

Halmos similarly highlights the "faith" (rather than the science) of the counsellors. In his view, the therapist's belief in the possibility of overcoming neurosis, of health triumphing over illness, is a secularized version of the priestly preoccupation with the struggle between good and evil.

It is, of course, true that a therapist, like any individual, does have a value system, an ethical position. And it is equally true that therapists have their own therapeutic goals, which may be more or less explicit. Freud at different times offered an optimistic view of these aims, "to love and to work", and a more pessimistic one—transforming "hysterical misery into common unhappiness". Roy Schafer, in his discussion of "the psychoanalytic vision of reality", sees a successful analysis as producing

> A more united, subjective self, one which has more room in it for undisguised pleasure, but also for control, delay, decisive renunciation, remorse, mourning, memories, anticipation, ideals, moral standards, and more room too for a keen sense of real

challenges, dangers and rewards in one's current existence. The childlike regression and nostalgia is reduced in influence. [Schafer, 1976]

Psychotherapy undoubtedly does embody an ethical system. This can perhaps best be seen as part of what the Rustins call the "religion of humanism" (Rustin & Rustin, 1984), which is anti-authoritarian and in which individual experience and satisfying reciprocity in personal relationships are highly valued. Within this overall humanist framework, there is considerable scope for the varying beliefs and interests of individual schools and approaches.

These different ethical assumptions are more important than is often recognized in determining an individual's choice of therapy. Given a choice, she will probably seek out a therapist and a therapy whose ambience is congruent with her own unconscious themes and needs. But a good analytic therapist will also look behind this choice for the way in which an individual's defences influence her choice of therapy, and might insist that, if therapy is to do its job properly, these should be brought into awareness in the course of treatment.

THE BELIEVER AND HER THERAPIST

A woman in her 40s stated at the first interview that it was very important that her therapist believed in God. She had had a period of profound depression at the age of 18 after her father, to whom she was very attached, had died suddenly. Soon afterwards she married a divorced man twenty years older than herself, who was now ill. They had been unable to have children. In the course of the interview she suddenly asked the therapist point-blank if he believed in God. Rather sheepishly he replied "not exactly". She did not take up the offer of therapy. Later she wrote to explain that she had gone into treatment with a psychotherapist who was also a priest, whom she had known previously.

It is debatable whether or not the therapist should have answered her question directly, especially in such a half-hearted way. A technical purist might have refused to answer and said instead, "You wonder if I believe in God?"; a naive therapist, like the one reported, might have said "yes" or "no", as the case may have been.

Another approach might have been to say: "I will answer you in a minute, but let's first explore why the question is so important to you." This might have uncovered a romantic attachment to the priest, for example, and her feelings of guilt about this, which might well in turn have connected with her similar special and secret relationship with her father and her depression after his death. One of the difficulties that psychotherapy presents is the existence of several *levels* of communication, each of which requires due attention. At a non-technical level, the patient's question was a perfectly valid precursor to the therapy, checking on the therapist's beliefs and orientation in a way that would help her decide if he was the kind of person she would like to work with. This, colloquially, could be called the "off the couch" level of therapy (C. Rycroft, personal communication). At another, unconscious, "on the couch" level, her question could have been an expression of her desperate need to find an everlasting father whom she felt she had irretrievably lost. The good therapist has, if possible, to recognize both levels and not to foreclose by either a premature, rejecting, or evasive response.

The next example shows how the therapist's beliefs, while maintaining only a background presence, can become important when they are used as a guide to the patient's underlying feelings and attitudes.

THE WOMAN WHO "DIDN'T CARE" ABOUT BOYFRIENDS

A depressed, unmarried, and childless woman in her late 30s sought help after splitting up with her boyfriend. During an assessment interview she spoke of how alone and miserable she felt, but denied that she was upset because of the break-up with her boyfriend—"boyfriends come and go", she said dismissively. Her male therapist saw this dismissal as a defence against feelings of disappointment and abandonment, and tried to link it with her account of a childhood in which her parents had several times been away for months at a time, leaving her in the care of nuns and aunts. This suggestion, too, she rejected quite angrily, saying that there was nothing particularly abnormal about her childhood, and that thousands of other children had survived worse. Sensing the beginning of a battle between them, the therapist became silent and wondered if he was wrongly imposing his own values on the patient by suggesting that the lack of continuity of parental care in childhood could be detrimental. What about the Spartans, or the Victorian middle classes? Did they not grow up

successfully without much mother-love? He then began to wonder if the patient had unconsciously invited him to impress his
ethical position on her, and if he, equally unconsciously, had responded to this invitation, and whether this could not have been a
repetition of some earlier relationship. He tried to translate this
moral transaction between them into terms of transference and
countertransference and suggested that perhaps she was particularly sensitive to being imposed upon by other people's values.
She confirmed this by saying how terrified she had been to let her
mother, who had a strict moral code which she attempted to
impose on all who encountered her, know that she was living
with the boyfriend without their being married. She went on,
tearfully, to consider why it was that her relationships with men
tended to break down, and to see how "sensitive" and angry she
became when she felt they were "imposing" on her and how this
contributed to driving them away.

This is a long way from Rieff's conception of the therapist as
moral pedagogue. The therapist had to check himself from becoming
a didactic moral proselytizer like the patient's mother. The therapist's
values are there, and, like the impact of the observer in Heisenberg's
Uncertainty Principle (in which the act of observation at an atomic
level inevitably affects what is observed), have to be taken into account; unlike religious dogmas, however, they are not imposed but,
rather, can be used to further the therapy. The basis of this is the
therapist's capacity for self-awareness and detachment from her own
values and responses, and her ability to use them to understand the
interaction between herself and the patient.

Psychotherapy does have its own values and commitments. Like
political liberalism, however, it does not attempt to impose any particular set of substantive values. This is because it takes as axiomatic
the importance of the individual patient's choice. The aim is for the
patient to be able, as a result of therapy, to discover and where
necessary create her own substantive value system. No doubt psychotherapists do exert considerable moral influence on their patients,
but they are required to be self-reflective about this and to examine
this influence in the light of transference and countertransference.

Rieff's and Halmos's attempts to re-translate psychoanalytic
theory and practice into a quasi-religious ethic misses, in our view,
the heart of what is special about analytic psychotherapy. Interesting

and sometimes illuminating parallels exist between, say, the findings of modern physics and Taoist philosophy, or between Darwinism and Lucretian biology; but to reduce one to the other or to conflate them would be absurd. The ideas of the unconscious and the workings of transference and countertransference, although they too have their historical prefigurings, are discoveries that are unique to psychoanalytic therapy and create ethical problems of their own kind.

The distinctive ethic of analytic therapy is based on two assumptions, one philosophical, the other technical. The first is the liberal belief in the value of autonomy and individual choice. Psychotherapy is, more than anything, about helping people to choose; *what* they choose (with certain exceptions, which are considered in chapter eight) is left to them. The second is the centrality of transference and countertransference. The dilemmas that patients bring to therapy, and the ethical issues that arise out of them, must not just be taken at face value but seen in a context of unconscious needs and desires, of residues of childhood feeling that, while they remain outside of awareness, reduce autonomy and choice in adult life.

The psychotherapist as parent

If psychotherapy requires the acknowledgement and acceptance of childhood feelings, should the relationship between therapist and patient be modelled on that between parent and child? Certainly the moral qualities required of the therapist are similar to those that a child might ideally expect from a parent or care-giver: the capacity to provide security and stimulus; empathy and firmness; containment and freedom. In the seventeenth century, Francis Bacon saw that children were "hostages to fortune". It is important that a would-be psychotherapist should also understand the grave responsibility of "taking on" a patient for therapy, and be prepared to be reasonably reliable, consistent, and available over prolonged periods.

As with parents and children, patients need different responses from therapists at different times. An infant requires undivided attention and flexibility, as may a very regressed patient; a toddler may need limit-setting and containment; adolescents need friendship and guidance. The therapist, too, has to be sensitive to the psychological maturity of the patient, and respond accordingly. Infants and small children need to be seen as special by their parents, to be perceived with what Margaret Mahler calls "the glint in the parent's eye" (Mahler, 1969). Later, this residue of parental narcissism can be burdensome and impede the development of autonomy and reality-testing. Children need to know that they are ordinary as well as special. Similarly, it is often helpful for depressed patients who doubt their own worth to feel that their therapists see them as special and unique. Later in therapy, this tendency on the part of therapists to see their geese as swans can lead to a prolonged dependency or a collusive mutual admiration which is counter-therapeutic.

An overriding rule of parenthood and therapy is that the parent or therapist should not use those in their care for their own needs. Sexual abuse of children by parents and sexual abuse of patients by therapists are extreme examples of this; but more subtle forms of reversal of need are common. The parent who is too emotionally dependent on a child is doing the child a disservice; therapists must guard against similar tendencies to ensnare patients into gratifying their own needs to feel indispensable, good, generous, kind, or admirable. A therapist may feel all of these things in the course of therapy, and therapists *are* entitled to job satisfaction and appreciation where due; but this should come from a job well done—from understanding, helping the patient to be able to communicate more freely and to become more emotionally autonomous—not from gratification based on unanalysed positive transference.

Although there are clear parallels between the parent–child relationship and the therapeutic relationship, there is one obvious difference. The patient is *not*, except in child psychotherapy, a child; and even in child psychotherapy the patient is not the *therapist's* child. The therapist rarely behaves towards the patient as a parent would towards its own child. As Talcott Parsons, a psychoanalytically trained sociologist, puts it:

> It is true that the father role is perhaps the most immediately appropriate *transference* role to a male analyst, especially if there is a considerable age differential. But when a son misbehaves a father reacts with anger and punishment, not affectively neutral "understanding". A father can also be called upon to help where a physician can legitimately refuse. It is precisely the *differences* from friendship and familial roles which are the most important levers for the psychotherapeutic process. [Parsons, 1951]

The patient is not a child: for therapy to work she must have an adult part, an "observing ego" that can understand and nurture the childlike part of herself. As Freud pointed out, where this observing ego is lacking, as in severe psychosis or in some forms of psychopathic disorders, analytic psychotherapy is unlikely to succeed: the patient may become dependent on the therapist but will be unable to use that dependency to achieve autonomy. Equally, the therapist is *not* a parent. She is temporarily an idealized parent, the parent whom the patient would like to have had. The process of psychotherapy could be seen as a movement from metaphor to simile: from "You *are* the father that I feared and hated" to "You are *like* a father that I *imagined* I feared and hated"; from "You *are* my ideal mother" to "You are *like* a good-enough mother". For this movement to occur, the therapist has *both* to evoke real feelings in the patient, based on real characteristics, *and* to be sufficiently different or detached from this reality for the patient to see it as a metaphor. A similar process takes place in theatre, where the actor must portray a character lifelike enough for disbelief to be suspended, but be able to take the bow with the rest of the cast at the end of the performance. This "role responsiveness" (Sandler, 1976) on the part of the therapist is essential, but its necessary fluidity contributes to the difficulty in defining the nature of the profession.

The psychotherapist as friend, lover, or advocate

According to Sandor Ferenczi, one of Freud's early followers, who advocated an "active" attitude on the part of the therapist, "the physician's love heals the patient" (Ferenczi, 1955). As with parenthood, while there are some similarities between loving friendship and the therapeutic relationship, there are also important differences. The therapeutic relationship lacks the essential *reciprocity* of friendship, its companionship, and the *mutuality* of lovers. Alice Miller develops the idea that the therapist is the patient's *advocate*: "I always regard myself as the advocate of the child in my patients; whatever they may tell me, I take their side completely. . . . I consciously identify with the mute child in the patient" (Miller, 1985). Miller is critical of orthodox psychoanalysis, which she sees as avoiding the patient's real pain by analysing it rather than identifying with it. At the same time, analytic therapy aims always to go beyond the patient's need for love or friendship towards a deeper understanding of why the need is there and of defensive uses to which patients may put their vulnerability.

Therapists on the whole do their patients a disservice if they fall into the trap of simply befriending them. Patients are then more likely to remain stuck in the therapeutic relationship than to "internalize" it in a way that enhances autonomy and hence their relationships generally. This point is brought out in the following example.

THE WOMAN WHO HAD EVERYTHING

A wealthy but unhappy woman in her early 30s sought psychotherapy. She "had" everything: a successful and charming husband, children, ample material possessions, artistic talent, interesting and glamorous friends, all of whom were "special" to her. But still she felt empty and miserable inside. She was the only child of a self-centred but indulgent mother, and an absentee and impotent father. She trailed a series of devoted professionals and tradespeople who helped her with the problems of her life: "her" bank manager, accountant, children's teacher, garage mechanic, builder, doctor. Each was subtly shaped by her flattery, her attention, her occasional seduction. Each served her loyally. Each was "possessed" by her, as the possessive pronoun suggested.

When her marriage finally broke up she decided to seek psychotherapeutic help. As before, she unconsciously assumed that her first task, if she was to be accepted, was to seduce her therapist into liking her. Only by seduction would he be blinded to her self-disgust, to her core feelings of dishonesty and unworthiness. It was only natural that she and he should be friends, she insisted. An atmosphere of mutual flattery and excitement built up. But then came difficulty and disappointment. A line was drawn around her blandishments. The therapist refused her invitations to exciting parties and concerts. He did not invite her to his home. He discouraged her attempts to befriend his daughter, whom she had met at a party. At the same time, the patient was not rejected. Her behaviour was seen positively in that it brought into the therapy the heart of her problem, namely her feelings of being unwanted and her desperate attempts to overcome them by seduction and manipulation; her self-indulgence as a continuation of her mother's indulgent neglect of her as a child; her search for a loving and non-impotent father; her wish to be "special" because she felt so ordinary and insignificant; her assertion of female power because of her disappointments in men.

The psychotherapist as doctor:
transference

This example takes us into the heartland of psychotherapy, where the ethical dilemmas associated with analytic therapy are at their starkest.

Many patients harbour a desire to be liked by their therapists, who may in turn be tempted to befriend a likeable but lonely client. Patients wish to know about their therapists' lives and families. Therapists may find it difficult to withhold such information, feeling that to do so is artificial and cold. As his ideas developed, Freud came to see his temptation to turn the therapeutic relationship into love or friendship as a central issue in treatment.

> If someone's need for love is not entirely satisfied by reality he is bound to approach every new person whom he meets with libidinal anticipatory ideas—and it is highly probable that both portions of his libido, the portion that is capable of becoming conscious as well as the unconscious one have a share in forming that attitude. . . . It is perfectly normal and intelligible thing that . . . this . . . should be directed to the figure of the doctor. [Freud, 1912b]

At first Freud saw transference—the carrying over of emotions, reactions, and attitudes from the past, which he likened to "stereotype plates", into present relationships—as a resistance, a nuisance that interferes with the progress of treatment. He then realized that transference contains in a living form the very difficulties in relationships which contributed to the neurosis. He saw too that, alongside positive transference, there are also negative feelings towards the therapist that are equally important to analyse. By construing the relationship as a friendship, this opportunity is missed. The therapist has, through transference, an opportunity to help patients identify and understand themselves. If patients can come to know about those parts of themselves of which they are unaware, they will be less in thrall to them.

The central ethical difficulties of analytic psychotherapy can be seen as arising out of two contrasting technical "rules". The "fundamental rule" insists that the patient allows as many intense feelings and desires as possible—including those directed towards the therapist—to come into consciousness. The "rule of abstinence" insists that the therapist does not attempt to gratify these desires and discourages the patient from prematurely doing so outside the therapy. "I shall take it as a fundamental principle that the patient's need and longing should be allowed to persist . . . in order that they may serve as forces impelling her to do work and make changes" (Freud, 1912b). A similar injunction applies to negative transference: "Cruel though it may sound, we must see to it that the patient's suffering, to a degree that is in some way or another effective, does not come to an end prematurely" (Freud, 1912b).

These two contrasting rules—the rule of allowing feelings to surface and the rule of abstinence—mean that the therapist, as Winnicott puts it, "is under strain in maintaining a professional attitude" (Winnicott, 1965). Both therapist and patient are encouraged to respond in a personal and emotive way, and yet not to act on these responses. The "strain" is relieved when the patient's feelings are seen in the context of transference. By interpreting transference the therapist helps the patient to see her feelings in therapy as metaphor for her problems outside therapy. In this way, resolutions arrived at in therapy can be generalized to help overcome difficulties in the outside world. By becoming part of the problem, therapy contributes to its solution.

Analytic therapy attempts, through the use of transference, to resolve the paradox arising from the need for intimacy if therapy is to succeed, and the equally important need for the therapist to find a non-intimate, neutral position from which to get some leverage on the patient's problem. By stepping back from friendship or love the therapist avoids the vicious circle in which the neurotic individual elicits responses that serve only to reinforce her neurosis. As Talcott Parsons puts it:

> There must be an "Archimedean place to stand" outside the reciprocities of ordinary social intercourse. This is precisely what the patterning of the therapist's role provides. Whether it is love or hate which the patient projects upon [her], [she] fails to reciprocate in the expected terms. [She] remains objective and affectively neutral. . . . The discrepancy between the transference reactions and the real role of the therapist provides one of the most important occasions for interpretations which can bring the patient to new levels of insight. [Parsons, 1951]

Countertransference

Parson's principle is a counsel of perfection; in practice it is not so easy to maintain both sensitivity and neutrality. A physician, before conducting a physical examination, will allow the patient to take her clothes off in private so as to minimize any sexual connotations, for physician or patient, of undressing. The psychotherapist is in a more difficult position. According to the "fundamental rule", she must avoid any attempts to suppress her own or her patients' feelings. The more defended she is, the less able is she to respond to the patient empathically, but the more she responds, the less able is she to retain a professional attitude.

The therapist is caught up in a powerful emotional field in which she must be both professional and friendly, but never merely a professional or a friend. A special responsibility is placed upon her. She has to be able to identify the emotional responses in herself that the patient's transference has aroused, and to be sufficiently integrated and healthy not to act on them, but to use them, via interpretation, to help the patient. These responses constitute the therapist's *countertransference*. Turning emotional response into interpretation, if it is done in a living and creative way and not mechanically, is always difficult. As James Strachey puts it:

> The giving of a mutative interpretation [that is, one which leads to change] is a crucial act for the analyst as well as for the patient and [she] is exposing [herself] to some great danger in doing so. . . . At the moment of interpretation the analyst is in fact deliberately evoking a quantity of the patient's . . . [primitive feelings] while . . . [they are] alive and unambiguous and aimed directly at [herself]. Such a moment must above all others put to the test [her] relations with [her] own unconscious impulses. [Strachey, 1934]

Opening oneself up to transference and countertransference requires a certain amount of moral fortitude on the part of the therapist. The temptation is towards avoidance—to talk about the patient's childhood, give priestly advice, make suggestions, respond in kind to offers of friendship or even seduction, or give "transference interpretations" in a defensive, rejecting, or clichéd way that merely distances the patient.

Winnicott, in the light of these temptations, sees the need for therapists to have their own therapy: "I am not saying that the analyst's analysis is to free him from neurosis; it is to increase the stability of character and maturity of the personality, this being the basis of our ability to maintain a professional relationship" (Winnicott, 1965).

Therapists are often severely tested morally by their patients. They have to be as open and sensitive as possible, but must not retaliate or pretend to be perfect, nor put their own wish to be seen as "good" before the patient's need to explore, attack, despair, and be reconciled.

By understanding the ethical problems that arise in therapy in terms of transference and countertransference, a therapeutic space is created in which the patient can explore feelings without the normal moral constraints of reciprocity and obligation. We have drawn an analogy between therapy and theatre. Just as the evil embodied, say, in the character of Iago, is not corrupting but confirmatory of a moral order, so in therapy the patient has an opportunity to see her "badness" as a necessary part of humanity, not as something that needs to be eliminated. When manifested in transference, "badness" is not an enacted evil but can be recognized as metaphorical. "Non-attachment" as an ethical ideal derived from Buddhism is a relevant stance for the psychotherapist (Holmes, 1996), who has to be able to see evil for what it is without either condoning or condemning it.

In summary, we have so far made three points in this chapter. First, we have argued that the tension between intimacy and professionalism, which exists to some extent in all professions, is particularly marked in psychotherapy, and psychotherapeutic intimacy is likely to impose considerable moral strain upon the therapist. Second, we have shown how understanding transference and countertransference enables this strain to be relieved, and that the reflexive technical use of the therapist's and patient's feelings and frailties also demarcates psychotherapy from other professions. Third, in consequence, the therapist has a special responsibility to conduct herself with the utmost moral delicacy, based on considerable self-knowledge and maturity.

With these points in mind, we now proceed to consider three commonly encountered quandaries within psychotherapy: the question of truth-telling, the issue of therapist self-revelation, and the problem of the proselytizing therapist.

Lies and truth in psychotherapy

Transference and countertransference require therapists to maintain a strong self-restraint. The therapist, like any other craftsman or professional, is in a sense a technician; but unlike a lawyer, a car mechanic, or a surgeon, she cannot readily make a split between the problem and the person. In psychotherapy the problem is the person. Freud liked to compare the analyst's detachment and incisiveness with that of a surgeon (Freud, 1912e). Unlike a surgeon, however, the therapist's field, and especially the unconscious, does not confine itself to one location, but permeates every aspect of behaviour and experience. This has significant ethical consequences for the therapist. If, in a shop or at a party, a surgeon meets a patient on whom she is soon to operate, there is no reason to suppose that this will affect the way that she conducts the operation. The implications of such a meeting between psychotherapist and patient are likely to be much greater, and the feelings aroused by such an encounter will need to be carefully considered.

All this puts the therapist in a peculiar position. On the one hand, she must reveal as little as possible about herself, while on the other she has responsibility to be honest and truthful. She must not deceive the patient, yet an atmosphere is created in which the patient may feel, because so little is revealed, that she is being insulated from the truth.

THE MISSING RING

A patient who, as a child, had always thought of himself as his mother's "little husband" and denied the importance of his parents' marriage, suddenly noticed his therapist's wedding ring. He was furious. "You never told me you were married", he complained. But the marriage and the ring were there all along. Only through the reticence of the therapist was the patient's transferential self-deception revealed to him.

The therapist has a responsibility not to lie but, at the same time, for there to be, in Burke's sense (rather than Sir Robert Armstrong's), "an economy of truth". As Freud put it:

Psychoanalytic treatment is founded on truthfulness. In this fact lies a great part of its educative effect and ethical value. It is dangerous to depart from this foundation. Anyone who becomes saturated in the analytic technique will no longer be able to make use of the lies and pretences which a doctor normally finds unavoidable; and if, with the best intentions, he does attempt to do so, he is very likely to betray himself. Since we demand strict truthfulness from our patients, we jeopardize our whole authority if we let ourselves be caught out by them in a departure from the truth. [Freud, 1912e]

Deception jeopardizes the therapeutic process in two ways. First, in the obvious sense that the therapist cannot be sure that she will not be found out, thus destroying the trust a patient must have in her for successful therapy; second, in the sense that deception would undermine the moral authority of a therapist whose work is predicated on the principle that people should face up to the truth about themselves, even if this is painful.

Any deceit, however apparently trivial, can have implications for the therapeutic process, especially because it is likely to be influenced by transferential forces. It is not important merely for the therapist to be truthful; the way in which the truth is presented and used as a guide to transference is crucial, as the following example illustrates.

THE THERAPIST WHO "FORGOT" TO WRITE

A therapist had forgotten that she had agreed to write a letter to a male patient's employer about the times of his therapy sessions. The patient asked in the next session if the letter had been sent. The therapist was tempted to say "yes"—after all she could send it off immediately after the session, and it was important that the patient did not lose faith in the therapist when so many other figures upon whom he depended had let him down in the past. But she then began to wonder why she had forgotten, and realized that she resented this request on the part of the patient, whom she felt should be able to face his employer without her backing. She then linked this with the patient's own resentment of those who had cared for him in the past (his parents had died when he was 7, and he had been brought up by well-meaning but neglectful foster-parents), and with his expression of this resentment through his helplessness and a view of life in which he was always let down. The therapist therefore admitted that she had forgotten, but tried to link these themes to it. This proved productive. The patient went on to reveal that he was very angry with his employer, who had promoted a colleague over his head, and this in turn led to memories from childhood of misery and exclusion when his foster-parents unexpectedly had a child of their own.

A prime responsibility of the analytic therapist is to understand her own countertransference, and her inevitable mistakes, in the light of the interaction between her own and the patient's psychic life. In this way transference and countertransference become reference points by which the ethical problems in therapy can be examined.

It was not forgetting to write a letter in itself that was important, but its meaning for the patient. The implication of this is that apparently trivial moral dilemmas are likely to be of significance, and so, for the space of the therapy, the therapist is required to maintain a special moral arousal. This in turn means that therapists must be able to examine their motives by the process of "internal supervision" (Casement, 1985) and through support and supervision from colleagues. The therapist suppresses some of her "normal" responses: she neither blames herself, nor lies, but tries to find the meaning of what happened. In this sense therapists can be seen as similar to poets: as Sir Philip Sidney put it, "the poet nothing affirmeth, and therefore nothing lyeth". At the same time, the therapist must not use this moral suspension as a means of evading responsibility by blaming the patient. In our example, it was important that the therapist admitted that she *was* remiss in not writing the letter (which should, perhaps, never have been agreed to in the first place), even if there were "good" countertransferential reasons for this. She must be honest, and search for meaning, but not at the expense of empathy. She must allow that both she and the patient will on occasion fail, and that out of this failure, if it is approached correctly, will come progress.

Self-revelation and opacity

The choice between candour and reticence is often especially difficult for the therapist when the issue is that of self-disclosure. Patients frequently complain of the one-sidedness of therapy. Therapists are often tempted to help their patients through some form of limited self-revelation, hoping that this will reassure an anxious patient that she is not as mad, abnormal, or different, as she imagines. The Jungian analyst and author Anthony Storr rather courageously describes how

> When I was young and inexperienced, a man once came to see me whose principal problem was intense guilt about masturbation. His sessions with me were progressing fairly well, when one day he suddenly asked me, just as he was about to leave the room, whether I had ever masturbated. Without thinking, caught off my guard, I answered "Yes". I never saw that patient again. What I ought to have said was something like this "What reply are you hoping for? Are you wanting me to say 'No' because someone who has never masturbated is an ideal to you?", and then explored this phantasy further. It would probably have emerged that he had never been able to imagine his parents as sexual beings, and that he had completely unrealistic notions about male sexuality in general; but my thoughtless admission clearly disillusioned him about me to such an extent that he felt I could be of no use to him. [Storr, 1979]

Storr's example is an extreme version of a common ethical pitfall for therapists who may feel forced to choose between technical "correctness" (non-revelation) and an appropriate human responsiveness, which, however, could be, as in Storr's example, counter-therapeutic. Seeing the situation transferentially takes the therapist off the horns of the technique/friendship dilemma because it enables her to remain neutral and to get in touch with the pain or anxiety that underlies the patient's need for love and friendship.

Storr's example shows how the therapist can be mistaken in putting friendship before therapy. It is equally true that to avoid common humanity can be persecutory and counter-therapeutic.

THE UNSMILING ANALYST

One analyst working with in-patients refused to smile or even say "Good morning" as he walked through his ward, on the grounds that it would "interfere with the transference"; as a consequence, his patients were so terrified when they encountered him that they appeared much madder than in fact they were.

R. D. Laing is especially insistent that in psychotic patients empathic resonance must take precedence over transference interpretation:

I had begun a session with a schizophrenic woman of twenty-five, who sat down in a chair some distance away from me while I was sitting half facing her in another chair. After about ten minutes during which she had not moved or spoken, my mind began to drift away on to my own private preoccupations. In the midst of these, I heard her say in a very small voice, "Oh, please don't go so far away from me". When the patient made this remark, one could respond in a number of ways. A possible comment that some psychotherapist might make would be, "You feel I am away from you." By this, one would neither confirm nor disconfirm the validity of her "feeling" that I was no longer "with" her, but would confirm the fact that she experienced me as away. . . . However, in my view, the most important thing for the therapist to do in such a situation is to confirm that the patient has correctly registered my actual withdrawal of my presence if she has correctly done so. There are many patients who . . . cannot trust other people, and yet they cannot trust their own "intuitions" either. . . . The only thing, therefore, that I could say to my patient was, "I am sorry". [Laing, 1960]

The ethical dilemma for the therapist, then, is whether to be open with the patient as she might be with a friend, or to maintain a strict professional detachment. There is no absolute rule that will tell the therapist when to be self-revealing, when to remain opaque. Therapeutic tact cannot be legislated for. Similar considerations apply to the question of whether to touch patients in therapy. Touch can at times be immensely reassuring, but equally it can be experienced by patients as seductive or invasive. As with self-revelation, most therapists would tend towards reticence, since the harmful consequences of too much intimacy are potentially greater than those of too much restraint. Too much reticence can, however, be potentially confusing and persecutory for patients, who are often much more aware of their therapist's state of mind than they are given credit for. A therapist who experiences a major bereavement in the course of therapy would do well to consider giving her patients at least an inkling of what has happened, since they are likely to realize that something is wrong anyway. In the end, she will have to rely on her therapeutic intuition about how much to tell. There is an apparent irrationality about the therapist having, ultimately, to rely on intuition, but analytic therapists tend to place great value on it so long as it is tempered by reason: "where id is, there ego shall be." The therapist needs, through training and self-discipline, to be as aware of her own responses as possible, and of the ways in which her "intuition" will inevitably be influenced by transference and countertransference. The force of transference is so great that mistakes are almost bound to be made. But, as Winnicott points out, like a parent a therapist need only be "good enough", not perfect, and therapy often progresses through mistakes.

THE DETECTIVE STORY

A young therapist was asked by a patient, "What do you do when you are depressed?" "Oh, go to bed with a good detective novel", he replied. "Ah, so you get depressed too", she said.

This spontaneous response was an abandonment of the conventional reticence of the therapist and could have obstructed the progress of the therapy. The patient professed that she was relieved to know that the therapist, like her, was capable of frailty, was not some superhuman being, but there was also a triumphant sense in her of having cut him down to size, of having acquired a weapon that made her feel less small and insignificant. While the therapist was technically wrong to have responded as he did, it may have had the positive effect of "holding" a very ambivalent patient in therapy. Eventually what emerged in her therapy was an intense competitiveness with men, originating in her parents' adoration of her brother, and a feeling of having been neglected as a child by parents who were so wrapped up in their own depression that they could not attend to her needs. Understanding this emerged slowly and painfully. Had the therapist not responded as a friend when she asked her question, and offered instead a transference interpretation, it is possible that the heart of the problem would have been reached by a quicker, more reliable, and more direct route, but equally the patient might have felt snubbed, unable to express her anger about this, and could have dropped out of therapy prematurely.

Proselytizing in psychotherapy

Earlier in this chapter we resisted Rieff's contention that psychotherapy is a form of secularized moral proselytizing. We argued that, rather than espousing any particular set of substantive values, psychotherapy tries to expose the psychological mechanisms that underlie different moral alternatives, and so help the patient to choose between them. In this, it is congruent with the liberal conception of individuality.

Liberals place great value on individual choice and autonomy. Believing in the worth of autonomy is itself espousing a value. However, liberals are opposed to forcing particular conceptions of a good life on people. Thus, psychotherapy and liberalism *do* have a moral viewpoint—that individuals should be free to make their own choices, at least to the extent that this does not harm other people's chances of doing the same. This may put psychotherapists in the ethically dubious position of forcibly telling their patients to "be autonomous", or of imposing what they see to be the obvious truth onto patients. Freud recognized the latter danger when he stated that interpretations should be made only when patients were half-way to discovering them for themselves.

Psychotherapists are certainly not immune from priggishness or an overbearing conviction of their own rectitude and importance. They have to find a way to remain true to their own substantive values, and at the same time to respect their patients' autonomy. We discuss some more extreme examples of this dilemma in the later chapters. Our next example illustrates how a therapist's *furor therapeuticus* may run away with her, with possibly harmful results for the therapy.

THE ARTIST'S HUSBAND

A man in his 50s sought help after his wife, an artist to whom he had been married for twenty-five years, committed suicide by drowning. He was referred to a supervisory therapist in a psychotherapy organization, who in turn referred him to a junior colleague. The bereaved man had decided to make a memorial catalogue of his wife's paintings, and this reparative project had greatly helped him with his grief. On the way to his tenth session he collected from a gallery one of her paintings, which was to be photographed. He felt worried that the picture might be stolen from his car and so brought it into the consulting-room. The picture, painted two years before his wife's death, was a Braque-like still life showing a table with a tablecloth, on which were two fish side by side on a dish, a yellow box of "Ship" matches, and, above, a picture-within-a-picture showing a peaceful rural scene with cows grazing.

The therapist immediately started to interpret the picture, which she said prefigured the artist's death. The fish looked uncomfortable together, she said, a sign that the marriage had been in difficulties; the tablecloth represented the sea, but there was no ship on the matchbox so the artist was already "drowning". The only peaceful part of the picture was the picture; only through art or death could she achieve peace.

The patient was furious. He complained that the therapist had no understanding of art: painting fish in that way was part of a twentieth-century artistic tradition; the box of matches was needed for its colour values, and putting a ship on it would have been distracting to the eye. He walked out of therapy, never to return.

There was certainly some truth in the therapist's interpretation of the picture. The artist may well have been struggling with depressive feelings at the time it was painted. But was the therapist right to introduce this retrospective analysis at this point? Was she not *imposing* a view of the picture which, however valid, was at variance with the patient's feelings at that moment?

The therapist's first duty must be to provide a secure frame or *containment* for the patient. This will be jeopardized, as in this case, if she uses her position to impose a view of reality on the patient, rather than helping him to find his own vision of the truth. The therapist must always use insights judiciously. The patient's need to be understood should take precedence over the therapist's need to make self-satisfying interpretations.

An awareness of transference might have led her to wonder whether, in addition to the common-sense reasons offered by the patient, there were not other unconscious, transferential, "on the couch" levels at which the meaning of bringing the picture should be considered. Perhaps he wanted to show the therapist how he wished his wife had not been "stolen" from him, leaving him with just pictures and a therapist; perhaps he wanted to explore his feelings of guilt and the drive to deal with these by making the catalogue. Had the therapist been in touch with her own countertransference, she might also have asked herself why it was so important for her to make a "brilliant" interpretation. Perhaps she was narcissistically using her patient because she wanted her supervisor to know how clever she was; perhaps she sensed the patient's need for an intelligent and creative woman and wanted to offer herself in this role; perhaps she felt rivalry towards the dead wife and wanted to diminish her idealized memory.

In this section, we have argued that therapists have a special moral responsibility to guard against their own self-righteousness and omnipotence. As one therapist put it, "Eighty per cent of the time I have no idea of what is going on between me and the patient." Keats's conception of "negative capability" captures the capacity to tolerate the uncertainty that is intrinsic to an activity aimed at enhancing autonomy. "Be autonomous", like "Be spontaneous", is only paradoxical if it is regarded as a direct order, intended to be directly obeyed. The painful intimacies of the therapeutic relationship push the therapist towards finding "answers", either through some definite explanation of the patient's pain, or by offering a substitute that will alleviate the effects of past deprivation. But the therapist has to position herself *alongside* the patient, neither pushing her from behind nor dragging her into pseudo-certainties. This autonomy-enhancing companionship does not, as Alice Miller puts it, "represent a 'corrective emotional experience' (for nothing can correct the past) but it does enable [her] to break through to [her] own reality and to grieve" (Miller, 1985).

Psychotherapy enhances autonomy by enabling an individual to choose more freely, in the sense of effectively pursuing the goals that she values, and by increasing her awareness of herself, her history, and her position in the world. Because psychotherapists are likely to believe strongly that these are desirable goals, they have a special responsibility to examine how countertransference may influence them to try to *impose* these views on their patients, and to be correspondingly vigilant against doing so.

Conclusion

As discussed in the first part of this book, the distinctive value of psychotherapy is that it enhances emotional autonomy. From the psychotherapeutic point of view, there are several important interconnected concomitants of autonomy, alongside the *essential* constituents mentioned above (the capacity to choose freely and to know and understand oneself, one's biography, and one's position in the world).

These include self-esteem and the capacity to form and sustain satisfying relationships. We do not claim that psychotherapy is the only route to autonomy. Normal psychological and social development, education, and other activities all make important contributions, but we see psychotherapy as unique both in its aims, specifically to enhance *emotional* autonomy, and in some of the means, including transference and countertransference, it uses to achieve this.

In this chapter we have tried to show how the pursuit of autonomy as an overt goal creates special problems for the analytic therapist as she walks a tightrope between the need to reach the patient's innermost thoughts and feelings and the necessity to maintain professional detachment. We have tried to show how she may deviate by over-involvement or too much detachment, and how the notion of transference acts like a tightrope-walker's pole, to counterbalance and so maintain her poise. The most important ethical safeguards in analytic psychotherapy, as we see it, are: first, the therapist's capacity to understand transference and countertransference; second, the safety net of her personal stability; third, her own therapy; finally, supervision.

Supervision

In several of the examples that we have given in this chapter, the therapist follows a series of steps:

1. She is confronted by a decision or question to which she is uncertain of the answer: shall I tell the patient about any religious beliefs? Shall I admit to not having written the letter?
2. An action then follows in which she may feel that she has made a "mistake".
3. She then, by a process of introspection, tries to understand what has happened between herself and the patient in terms of transference and countertransference.
4. With the help of this introspection, the "mistake" can then often be retrieved and/or lead to a deepened understanding of the nature of the patient's difficulties.

In these ethical tight corners, the therapist is often forced into some kind of action, but with the aid of introspection she can also reflect upon what is happening. To do this, the therapist has to be able to sustain a benign splitting, in which one part of herself is observing and trying to understand this process. It is when the therapist is unable to be "self-containing" in this way that ethical difficulties are most likely to arise. The most immediate safeguard against such failures of self-observation is the process of supervision by a third party. By focusing on what is going on *between* patient and therapist rather than *within* the patient, and by allowing the therapist to recall her emotions in tranquillity, supervision can act as a counter-weight to the powerful feelings generated in the therapist by being in a situation of such intimacy with her patient. This may be compared with the advantages of two care-givers in bringing up young children. Children of parents who have to face the intense demands of child-rearing on their own may be at risk. A similar risk befalls the patients of a "one-parent" therapist.

In our view, supervision should be an essential part of an ethically acceptable psychotherapy, and patients have a right to expect that all therapists will have access to supervision. The process of supervision helps overcome the technical and moral difficulties that result from the lack of absolute rules in therapy. There may be no therapeutic "ten commandments", but supervision can ensure, despite this moral fluidity, that therapists maintain an ethical attitude. It can also help the therapist to demarcate the boundaries of therapy, and so differentiate those issues that belong "in" the therapy and can be resolved through understanding and interpretation; those issues that lie on the boundary and need to be established in the therapeutic contract; and those that belong outside and need extra-therapeutic responses. The latter possibility is illustrated by the next example, in which the therapist could be accused, like Nero, of fiddling while Rome burns.

THE GROUP AND THE FIRE

A group therapy session was taking place on the fifth floor of a hospital building. The fire alarm began to ring. Since there were frequent fire practices and false alarms, the therapist continued with the session unperturbed and, indeed, interpreted the group's increasing restlessness and anxiety in terms of a forthcoming holiday break. It was only when the smoke began to billow under the door that therapy was finally abandoned and the group was hastily evacuated down the emergency fire escape.

Another, probably apocryphal, anecdote illustrates how transferential understanding may not be equal to a situation where action rather than words is called for.

THE APOCRYPHAL MURDERER

A patient announced to his therapist that he would not be coming to his next session. When asked why, the patient said that he intended to shoot his boss on that day. The therapist responded: "Do what you like with your free time, but don't use it as an excuse for not coming to therapy."

This anecdote is given a special poignancy by the Tarasoff case (see chapter eight), in which a psychotherapy patient actually carried out a murder threat, and the therapist was subsequently sued by the victim's parents. At the beginning of this chapter we characterized *ethical* problems as ones to which there is no obvious technical solution. The dilemma faced by a therapist who has a patient threatening violence against another is a case in point.

Therapists have special responsibilities towards their patients, but they also have responsibilities towards the community in which they live. We have tried to show in this chapter that many of the ethical dilemmas that arise in therapy can be better understood if a transferential perspective is adopted. If the psychotherapeutic relationship were merely a form of friendship, for example, then what *would* be wrong with therapists having sex with their patients? By seeing it as analogous to incest and recognizing the damage that may result from incest, an apparently arbitrary external prohibition takes on psychological meaning. But therapists do not just talk to their patients. They *do* sometimes, in spite of their awareness of all its dangers, form sexual relationships with them. And patients do sometimes act irresponsibly, dangerously towards themselves and others.

Protection of patients *and* the public will be a major issue if, as we have proposed, psychotherapy is greatly expanded. In the remaining chapters, we discuss some of the ethical dilemmas that arise from particular types of therapy and put forward proposals about how psychotherapists as a body should address them, especially concentrating on those problems that do not obviously admit of a technical solution.

CHAPTER SEVEN

Moral dilemmas
within psychotherapy

P sychotherapy matters because *autonomy* matters. The crucial evaluative assumption on which the case for psychotherapy depends is that personal autonomy has intrinsic worth as a part of human well-being. As we argued in chapter three, this assumption cannot be proved, but it is, we maintain, central to the liberal democratic tradition and is widely accepted, even by many critics of psychotherapy. Closely connected with this belief in the great importance of autonomy are principles of respect for the individual, encapsulated in statements such as "Never treat a person simply as a means to an end", "Every person is entitled to the maximum liberty compatible with a like liberty for all", and "Treat other people as you would have them treat you". The connection arises from the belief that it is people's capacity for autonomy which gives them *dignity*, by virtue of which they should be treated with individual respect.

Principles of respect are inextricably linked to a recognition of the intrinsic value of individual autonomy. This means giving special consideration to what individuals autonomously want, and to the promotion of their autonomy through time. It does not mean that nothing else matters, but rather that, for example, where there is a conflict between what people autonomously want and what would spare them pain, including mental pain, one should be prepared sometimes to give greater weight to the autonomy than to the avoidance of pain.

Hinshelwood (1995), arguing from a Kleinian perspective, makes a similar point in his critique of the simplistic use of the notion of autonomy in psychotherapy. He argues that autonomy is a concept that can only be applied to the conscious part of the self, and that the aim of psychotherapy is better seen as that of *integration* of discordant parts of the self, especially those unconscious aspects that are manifest in splitting and projection. However, the idea of emotional autonomy put forward here seems consistent with Hinshelwood's perspective, since we have argued that in order to become emotionally autonomous a person needs to get in touch with parts of herself of which she was previously unaware. This self-knowledge may be achieved through interpretation and insight in the analytic tradition, or by the self-monitoring of automatic thoughts and assumptions that characterize cognitive-behavioural treatments.

Many difficult moral dilemmas of ordinary life stem from situations where there is a conflict between what someone currently wants and what, in the view of a would-be helper, appears to be in her long-term interests. The helper can see the possibility of a more integrated, emotionally autonomous life, while the sufferer is caught up in a partial view of herself and her situation. But it may not be obvious what a respecter of autonomy should do in such cases, especially when the promotion of a person's long-term autonomy may require the overriding or even manipulation of present wants (for a general discussion of this kind of dilemma, see Lindley, 1986). Most other moral dilemmas arise out of cases where it is necessary to mediate conflicts of interest *between* people. In this chapter, we are primarily concerned with dilemmas that arise from conflicts within a patient, between short- and long-term autonomy. In the next chapter, we consider dilemmas arising from possible conflicts between a therapist's responsibilities to her patients and those towards other members of the community.

Professional relationships create special kinds of obligation and responsibility. Lawyers, for example, have a special obligation to seek justice for their clients; doctors to promote the health of their patients; and psychotherapists to promote the emotional autonomy of their patients.

The moral problems to do with a conflict between what a person wants or chooses and what a would-be helper thinks is good for her are heightened in the psychotherapeutic relationship for two reasons. The first is well captured by Sir John Foster in his *Enquiry into the Practice and Effects of Scientology*:

> Those who feel they need psychotherapy tend to be the very people who are most easily exploited: the weak, the insecure, the nervous, the lonely, the inadequate, and the depressed, whose desperation is often such that they are willing to do and pay anything for some improvement of their condition. [Foster, 1971]

The second—closely related, but different—is that the psychotherapeutic relationship itself creates a temporary dependency of the patient upon the therapist. As was pointed out in chapter six, the therapist–patient relationship has important similarities to that between child and adult. Just as children need special protection which is not available to adults, so psychotherapy patients, even if they are not children, may also need protection—against exploitation or abuse by unscrupulous or incompetent therapists.

The selection of dilemmas that we discuss in this chapter are illustrative of both the complexity and the range of moral problems that are the inevitable accompaniments of a psychotherapy service. Some are special problems for certain types of therapy, others apply to special circumstances in which therapy may be practised, and yet others apply to all therapies and all therapeutic situations.

Deception and manipulation in psychotherapy

To *deceive* is to get a person to form a belief or impression that the deceiver herself does not hold. Deception includes bare-faced lies, but also subtler ways of conveying a false impression. To *manipulate* a person is to treat her instrumentally, as an object of the manipulator's purposes rather than as an autonomous agent. From a moral point of view, deception and manipulation are closely connected: deception is a common form of manipulation, and the essential immorality of both is that they are inconsistent with respect for individual autonomy. Deception and manipulation are a direct assault on individuals' control over their own lives. Since, as we have claimed, psychotherapists have a special responsibility to protect and promote their patients' autonomy, one might expect that manipulation and deceit would be anathema to therapists and completely excluded from therapy. Freud, as we pointed out in chapter six, regarded honesty between therapist and patient as essential for psychoanalysis.

But most general rules have exceptions. Although deceit and manipulation are wrong in themselves, there are occasions when they might be justifiable. A favourite philosophers' example is the case of someone confronted by a murderer who asks which way his intended victim has fled. The person asked knows where the victim has gone, and the murderer will not (on pain of murdering the person being questioned) allow her to evade the questions. Should she lie?

Immanuel Kant argued that even in these circumstances it would be wrong to lie, since the duty of honesty is strict and formal, not resting on appeal to consequences (Kant, 1798). Kant claimed that in such a case the honest informer would not be responsible for the victim's subsequent murder, this being the responsibility of the murderer, and that a single dishonest statement constitutes an assault on the whole framework of morality. Kant is right to point out that in ordinary life a decision to speak truthfully to someone should not be contingent on a calculation of the consequences of lying on that occasion. But his view of responsibility is problematic, since the informer *is and knows she is* in a position to make the difference between the victim's escaping and her being murdered; and Kant's conclusion that it would be wrong to lie to the murderer is rejected by almost everyone, philosophers and non-philosophers alike.

To manipulate or deceive someone is to treat that person, in Kant's phrase, "as a means to an end" rather than as an "end in himself". Nearly everyone would agree that it is wrong to manipulate or deceive either gratuitously or for base motives—for example, to take advantage of an innocent victim for one's own enrichment. Dilemmas usually arise on occasions when honesty and straightforwardness conflict with other values, most frequently, as in the example, with benevolence. The philosopher's example is deliberately extreme, perhaps so extreme that for most people the situation of the informer would not constitute a dilemma at all. It is obvious to most people that it would be right to lie to the murderer. There are, however, many occasions within private and public life where the possibility of deception poses a genuine moral *dilemma*. Examples include white lies to children, doctors deceiving patients in order to spare them pain, and politicians lying about the economy in order to prevent a run on the currency. For an excellent general discussion of the dilemmas of deception, see Bok (1978).

One might, in the light of the above, suppose that there could be occasions within psychotherapy when manipulation or deceit would be justifiable—for example, in an emergency, as in the story of the Zen monk living in a village by the sea who, knowing of an imminent tidal wave, but failing to persuade the villagers to escape, tells them that their rice fields on the hills are on fire. They rush up to see, and, through deception, are saved. But some therapies go far beyond using deceit and manipulation only occasionally, in emergencies—in spite of Freud's strictures about honesty, they unashamedly make use of manipulation and deceit, apparently as an integral part of the therapy. Is this morally acceptable?

The clearest example is the use of "paradoxical" interventions, most commonly in family therapies. A paradoxical intervention is one in which apparently absurd, incongruous, counter-therapeutic, or even blatantly false statements are used to produce a beneficial therapeutic result. A common example is *prescribing the symptom*, where a patient might be warned by the therapist about the dangers of abandoning a pattern of behaviour that the therapist is seeking to change. The ultimate aim of the prescription is precisely to jolt the patient into changing in the ways the prescription warns against. To an outsider this sounds like the sort of manipulation and deception that is hard to reconcile with respect for the patient as an autonomous individual. As such, one might suppose that it would be justifiable only in emergencies.

However, there are influential and respected therapists who not only employ these techniques, but deny that they raise any ethical problems. Consider, for example, this argument from Watzlawick and his co-workers, a group of leading American family therapists who see no moral objection to outright manipulation of patients by therapists:

> Sincerity has lately become a catchword, a hypocrisy in its own right, associated in a murky way with the idea that there is such a thing as a "right" view of the world—usually one's own view. It also seems associated with the idea that "manipulation" is not only bad, but can be avoided. Nobody, unfortunately, has ever explained how this can be done. It is difficult to imagine how any behavior in the presence of another person can avoid being a

communication of one's own view of the nature of one's relationship with that person and how it can, therefore, fail to influence
that person. . . . The problem, therefore, is not how influence and
manipulation can be avoided, but how they can best be compre-
hended and used in the interest of the patient. [Watzlawick,
Weakland, & Fisch, 1974]

These writers seem to be saying that therapists should not regard
themselves as under any obligation to be honest with their patients
about what is going on in the therapy, or to avoid manipulation.
Sincerity is not a problem, apparently, since there is no such thing as
a "right" view of the world; manipulation is not morally problematic,
since it is unavoidable in any human encounter. What a therapist
says to, or does with, her patient should therefore be determined
exclusively by strategic considerations of what is in the patient's interests.

The relativist's claim about there being no "right" view of the
world is highly contentious, and even if it were true, would not
license deception—where the deceiver deliberately misleads her
victim. The claim that manipulation is inevitable simply rests on a
confusion between "influencing" and "manipulating". They are quite
different, since manipulation is, of its essence, intentional and surrep-
titious. For further discussion of Watzlawick's argument, see Collier
(1987) and Lindley (1987).

Watzlawick et al. deny the existence of a serious moral dilemma
that therapists, especially those who espouse paradoxical approaches,
ought to face. But for those who profess a belief in the importance of
autonomy, to treat manipulation in this cavalier way is to be guilty
of rank hypocrisy. Furthermore, there is a danger, in those therapies
that rely on paradox, that the therapist will lose sight of the fact that
she is working in an intimate way with someone whose interests may
be directly harmed by manipulation and deception, whether or not
they are discovered.

There are two forms of objection to manipulation and deception:
direct (they are wrong in themselves), and indirect (they lead,
whether intended to or not, to harmful consequences). As far as the
direct objections to deception and manipulation are concerned, they
stem from a principle of respect for autonomy. If this is true, then,
from the point of view of an ethical concern for autonomy, they
should not be objected to when resort to them actually *enhances* the
autonomy of the alleged victim of the deception.

It could be, for example, that the only way of enabling a particular patient to regain, or even develop for the first time, an acceptable level of autonomy, is to use a somewhat manipulative strategy. There are occasions where a patient may be locked into a destructive pattern of behaviour from which she cannot escape because of anxiety about the possibility of failure. Under these circumstances, concern for the patient's autonomy could rightly lead a therapist to use manipulative strategies to release the patient from her self-imposed prison, and enable her to change and thus become more autonomous and acquire greater self-esteem.

Consider the following example of the work of a British family therapist, Brian Cade (1979). He was treating a woman who had been regarded as "inadequate" and "chronically depressed" for several years. Previous attempts at psychotherapy had not worked, and she reached a state where she rarely got up before noon. When she was up, she spent most of the day lazing around on the sofa, complaining of a variety of ailments. Cade visited her for the first time shortly before Christmas, she having expressed a dread of Christmas and reluctance to see yet another therapist.

> I expressed considerable concern over her state of health, saying that I was extremely worried about her. I expressed shock at how early she was attempting to get up each day for a woman in her condition. Under no circumstances should she be up before at least three o'clock in the afternoon; if necessary she should remain in bed all day. As for housework and cooking, these were to be done by the rest of the family; the woman was solemnly warned that she was not to attempt such tasks. I went on to express admiration at the brave attempt made by the woman to be a good wife and mother. I, however, agreed with her decision not to tax herself by trying to make something of the festive season. [Cade, 1979]

According to Cade the woman was up at 8.30 the following morning, tidied the house thoroughly, and went out to do the Christmas shopping. The family had the best Christmas for years.

In this case the therapist deliberately told the patient a falsehood—that he was shocked at how *early* she was getting up in the morning. He then gave her a paradoxical command—to carry on behaving the way she had been, only more so.

There are two reasons for thinking that this apparent use of deception and manipulation by the therapist was not wrong. First, the aim and result of Cade's intervention was to enable the woman to escape from the rut of lethargy and depression from which she had been suffering for a considerable time, and from which she wanted to escape. Given that she did want to find a way out of her lethargy and depression, and had tried more direct methods which failed, it does not seem that Cade's paradoxical intervention was in itself inconsistent with a proper respect for his patient. Nothing in the intervention was inconsistent with the therapist's taking seriously the fact that his patient was someone with her own projects and values, who should be respected in the same way as anyone else. Indeed, patient and therapist here shared and achieved a common goal.

Second, it is not clear how the expression of shock and the paradoxical commands would have been taken and were intended to be taken by the patient. The communication of information requires the speaker to intend that the listener acquire a new belief. Attempted communicative manipulation or deception typically requires that the speaker tries to induce within the listener a belief that the speaker does not believe to be true. In this case, it is by no means clear that Cade made, or intended to make, his patient believe that he was genuinely shocked that she rose as early as midday. Nor is it clear that he really made, or intended to make, her believe that he thought her well-being required her to stay in bed even longer and to do no housework. In fact what we have here is not so much *deception*, as a skilful use of irony and sarcasm.

A good therapist will be able at least to suggest what her real aims are, by the judicious use of tone of voice, humour, and gesture. The aim of a paradoxical intervention is to disrupt a rigid pattern of thought or behaviour. It is usually, indeed essentially, ambiguous. In this case, the patient knew that an objective of the therapy was that she should start getting up early and living an active life, and yet here was the therapist telling her to do the opposite. The intervention put the patient in a position where if she obeyed the injunction literally she would be accepting the authority of the therapist, which she had hitherto rejected, whereas if she disobeyed, as she in fact did by getting up early, she would be manifesting autonomy and escaping from her disabling conditions. For a further discussion, see Holmes (1985).

A successful therapist, like a successful spouse, has to be adept in the art of tact. What one says may have meanings at different levels, and it may be impossible simultaneously to say what is true at all levels. Sometimes saying what is literally true may communicate a falsehood at a deep level, and sometimes expressing a literal falsehood may be the only way of communicating a more significant truth. Spouses who insist on telling each other about all their sexual fantasies do not necessarily enhance their marriage. On the other hand, if they cannot share their intimate feelings, or if they lead a double life, their relationship is in a bad state. In cases where the communication of one truth will convey a false impression, what is important is to convey the more important truth, even if this is at the cost of conveying a literal, though less significant, falsehood. In such a situation, the most one could do would be to minimize distortion of one's true beliefs. Between indiscriminate openness and deliberate dishonesty lies a whole spectrum of cases, and therapists should beware lest warranted tact turn into unwarranted manipulative deception. Dishonesty may be the lesser of two evils, but it is an evil nonetheless, and always requires a specific justification.

The problem of tact and deception is one that confronts doctors in charge of the sick and the dying, and it may appear that the psychotherapist's dilemma is really just like the doctor's; however, this would not be entirely correct. The doctor's prime responsibility to the patient is to cure or manage the patient's disease, and the deception is normally extrinsic to the treatment. The commonest occasion for deception is where the doctor either lies about, or deliberately fails to reveal, the true seriousness of the patient's illness. The normal motivation for this is to spare the patient pain. The patient's autonomy is sacrificed because it is thought that sparing her pain is, in these circumstances, more important. A more complicated situation arises when the doctor has reason to believe that the patient does not want to be told the truth about her condition. Here there is a dilemma *not between autonomy and pain relief, but between concern for different aspects of patient autonomy.* The doctor who respects the patient's *autonomy* by going along with her wishes might be refusing to promote her overall autonomy by not "forcing" her to face up to her actual situation; self-deception and ignorance are themselves forms of heteronomy. In such a situation, it is far from clear whether respect for the patient's autonomy should induce the doctor to comply with her wishes, or to override her wishes and tell her the truth.

More worrying than Cade's ironic suggestion to the woman who did not get up in the morning is the use, in therapy, of full-blooded deception, where the therapist succeeds in inculcating a false (though therapeutically useful) belief in a patient. The therapist contemplating a paradoxical intervention that uses actual deception is not faced with an autonomy versus pain-reduction dilemma, but with a problem of what respect for autonomy requires. The therapist lies to or manipulates the patient in order to enable the patient to become more autonomous. But why should this be a dilemma? Should the therapist not simply aim for whatever strategy offers the best chance, in the long run, of maximizing the patient's autonomy overall?

Given the enormous benefits that a patient can gain from therapy, it may seem that a little deception here and there is not significant and is a small price to pay for successful therapy, and that manipulation and deception are not a serious problem within psychotherapy. This brings us to the indirect objection to the use of deceit and manipulation: they have harmful consequences. To be deceived may in itself be a way of being harmed, as is explained by Thomas Nagel (1979). To have significant false beliefs itself constitutes a lack of autonomy. In evaluating individuals' overall autonomy, it is necessary to examine not only how their actual conduct relates to their aims, but also how dependent their emotional stability is on false beliefs.

There is a need to protect patients from therapists who take too cavalier an approach to manipulation. Cade, for example, who accepts Watzlawick's argument about sincerity, writes the following:

> I never explain the way in which a paradox works to an individual or a family even after its use has produced a desired change. Understanding or insight is not seen as a prerequisite for change nor necessary during or after change. [Cade, 1979]

It is no doubt true that, in many cases, understanding and insight are not a prerequisite for removing undesirable symptoms. Cade says that they are also not necessary *during or after change*. To assess this claim, one has to ask: necessary *for what?* Without insight and understanding a person is *ipso facto* less in control of her life. Furthermore, without insight and understanding, a person may be less well able to avoid relapse when difficulties occur in new circumstances.

If it were established that a given manipulative or deceptive intervention would promote the patient's overall autonomy, one could argue that this should silence any objections to such interventions which are based on an appeal to the value of autonomy. However, the precise effects of any given intervention are always unpredict-able. Any intervention, or indeed decision not to intervene, is effec-tively a gamble—a gamble that is, one hopes, the best for the patient. What seems wrong with even benevolent manipulations and deceptions is that the patient may want to be in control of her own gambles, to take her own risks, rather than be manipulated into situ-ations. For this reason, it makes a crucial difference whether or not the patient has genuinely consented to subject herself to the kind of treatment in question. If I go to the theatre, there is a sense in which I am agreeing to be taken in by the actors. Their performance and "deception" may be manipulative, but I am willingly manipulated in order properly to enjoy the play. It would be quite different if I had paid to see a comedy but was subjected instead to a frightening murder mystery. Similarly, if a patient enters family therapy aware of the fact that as part of the therapy she may be subjected to paradoxi-cal analyses and commands, then when she is subjected to them, this could be consistent with her ultimately being responsible for taking her own gambles. The manipulation is part of an overall strategy that she, the patient, has chosen.

Here, apparently unethical conduct is justified in part by its end—greater emotional autonomy overall—and in part by the supposition that the patient has, at least implicitly, given consent to the treatment. Suppose that a course of psychotherapy would result in a patient overcoming a debilitating neurotic disorder and becoming more in control of her life. If she chooses to enter into the therapy, knowing that this might entail being subjected to paradoxical techniques, the subsequent use of paradox for the agreed purpose is not inconsistent with respect for her autonomy, although this might present the tech-nical difficulty that knowing one is being subjected to paradox is likely to weaken the therapeutic impact of the paradox. There are two main ethical issues here: ensuring that gratuitous manipulation and deception are kept to a minimum, and seeing that where paradoxical techniques—which are *prima facie* an assault on the patient's auton-omy—are going to be used, the patient has genuinely consented. But how far does morality require a therapist to go in ensuring that her patients' consent to the therapeutic interventions they will receive is genuine?

The problem of informed consent

There is a vast literature in medical ethics on the subject of informed consent (see, for example, Appelbaum, Lidz, & Meisel, 1987). Does informed consent pose special problems for psychotherapy? With the exception, perhaps, of behaviour therapy, it is not in general possible to impose psychotherapy upon a completely unwilling subject, since therapy requires the cooperation of the patient. When someone agrees to have any form of psychotherapy her agreement may, however, be based on ignorance or a misunderstanding of what the therapy entails. Ensuring that consent to invasive or manipulative therapies is genuine and informed poses a serious moral dilemma for therapists. In some ways, the problem may be likened to that of doctors who require consent before performing an operation.

Doctors: a similar case?

If a doctor performs an operation on a patient without that patient's consent, the doctor is liable for the tort of battery. Except in emergencies—say, where an unconscious patient requiring immediate surgery is brought into a casualty ward—it is a legal as well as a moral offence to invade someone's bodily integrity without securing her agreement in advance. But just what does a patient have to consent to? In the case of *Devi v. West Midlands Area Health Authority* in 1980, a surgeon, during a dilation and curettage operation for which the patient had consented, discovered that the patient had a ruptured uterus. Acting, as he thought, in her best interests, he immediately performed a hysterectomy, obviously without her specific consent, while she was still anaesthetized for the dilation and curettage. The health authority was found liable for the battery committed by the surgeon. Although the patient had consented to surgery, and although the hysterectomy was most likely in her best interests, she had not consented to it, and without this consent the doctor should not have performed the operation.

But mere consent to a procedure may not count for much if the consent is not genuine. A doctor is under an obligation to explain to her patients, at least in broad terms, the nature of any proposed invasive surgery. In English law, consent is taken to be genuine provided that the practitioner has explained "in broad terms the nature of the procedure which is intended" (*Chatterton v. Gerson* [1981] 1 All ER 257, *per* Bristow J.), and "It is only if the consent is obtained by *fraud* or *misrepresentation* of the *nature* of what is to be done that it can be said that an *apparent* consent is not a true consent" (ibid.).

If a doctor explains in broad terms the nature of a procedure, but fails to spell out adequately the attendant risks and the likely benefits of alternative treatments, in English law she is, at most, guilty of the tort of negligence. Here, consequential damage has to be established, whereas battery is actionable *per se*.

In English law the test of whether or not the information about a procedure provided to a patient is sufficient is determined by the "reasonable body of medical opinion" test laid down in the case of *Bolam v. Friern Hospital Management Committee* ([1957] 2 All ER 118). Except in extreme circumstances, a doctor will not be held negligent for failing to warn a patient in sufficient detail of the risks of a procedure if her practice is in line with a substantial body of responsible medical opinion. In *Sidaway v. Royal Bethlem Hospital Governors* ([1985] 1 All ER 643), a surgeon performed spinal surgery on a patient, aimed at removing quite serious neck pains. He had, prior to surgery, informed her of the slight risk of "nerve damage": there was a slight risk (less than 1 per cent) of the operation causing paralysis, even if performed with all due care and skill. In the event, in spite of the skill of the surgical team, Mrs Sidaway was paralysed down her left side. The surgeon was held not to have been negligent in failing to inform her properly, since his actions were in line with the common practice of a substantial body of medical opinion.

In North America, by contrast, a legal doctrine of "informed consent" has developed. In the District of Columbia case of *Canterbury v. Spence* ([1972] 464 F 2d 772) for example, the following test was laid down for disclosing risks. A risk is required to be disclosed

> When a reasonable person, in what the physician knows or should know to be the patient's position, would be likely to attach significance to the risks or cluster of risks in deciding whether or not to forgo the proposed therapy. [ibid, at 787]

There is disagreement between the American and British courts over whether or not a "prudential patient" test such as that employed in parts of the United States is practicable. In the Sidaway case, for example, Lord Bridge claimed that the introduction of such a test would lead to too much uncertainty in the administration of the law.

What is clear, however, is that there is a big difference between consent that is "genuine" in the English sense, and what an ordinary citizen would call "genuine informed consent". If we leave out the practical legal difficulties of enforcement, the American conception has much to commend it from a moral perspective which takes autonomy seriously.

Doctors should aim to ensure that their patients are informed of relevant considerations before being asked to consent to invasive surgery. In general, this means telling the patient in broad terms of the nature of the treatment, picking out those elements of it that are likely to be of most interest to her in making up her mind whether or not to have the treatment, providing her with information about the risks attendant on the treatment, and informing her of alternative treatments. To secure consent in the absence of such information is to deny the patient the opportunity to make an autonomous decision about which treatment option to pursue.

Apart from the problem of time, there are two reasons why doctors are reluctant to provide their patients with this kind of information: to do so might cause a patient to reject a genuinely beneficial treatment, or, it might give the patient needless anxiety.

Special complications of psychotherapy

In certain important respects, psychotherapeutic treatment is similar to medical treatment. There is typically an "informational inequality" between patient and expert, and in the case of some therapies the patient may be subjected to invasions of autonomy which would normally require consent. In therapies using paradox, for example, a patient may be deceived and manipulated; in behaviour therapy, a patient may be subjected to a potentially degrading regime of reward and punishment; in Gestalt therapy, a patient may be subjected to harsh and painful criticism by other members of her group. The invasions of the psyche which psychotherapy often entails may be at least as serious as the physical invasions of medical treatment for which consent is required. On the other hand, psychotherapists, like doctors, may wish to protect their patients from unnecessary anxiety about a treatment that is in a patient's interests, and they may fear that too detailed an explanation may cause a patient to reject treatment on irrational grounds.

However, there are ways in which psychotherapy generates its own special problems concerning informed consent. In manipulative therapies, for example, a full and frank discussion of the techniques to be employed might render them ineffective. Suppose a therapist says to a patient, "Part of this therapy employs the technique of paradox. In other words, during the therapy I shall from time to time ask you to behave in just the ways that we all want you *not* to behave in." If this is explained in great detail to the patient, the effect of the paradoxical intervention may well be lost, since the patient may all too readily think: "This is obviously just a paradoxical intervention, I'm not going to be fooled by that." Analytic therapy, as we have seen, works mainly through free association and the analysis of transference. Both require spontaneity, which may be inhibited by the therapist explaining in too much detail, before therapy begins, how it is intended to work.

Related to this is the problem that it is very difficult to understand, even if someone tries to explain, how a therapy works, unless one has experienced it first-hand. An attempted explanation, although literally true, might well give a patient a misleading impression.

Another difficulty is that whereas the precise outcome of psychotherapy is, unlike the outcome of a medical procedure, almost impossible to predict, a full expression of this uncertainty to a patient contemplating therapy may undermine the therapy's chances of success, by falsely communicating a lack of confidence on the part of the therapist that it will be beneficial.

Furthermore, there is the serious problem that psychotherapy patients are more likely than, say, patients for surgery to suffer from emotional disturbance, which itself could vitiate the rationality of their decision-making. Someone who is seriously confused may, prior to therapy, not be able to consider dispassionately an account of the treatment and its alternatives.

There certainly are, then, formidable obstacles in the way of therapists ensuring that their patients have given informed consent prior to treatment. This puts therapists in a position of ethical hazard, since in such a situation it may be tempting to think, "Since fully informed consent is impossible, or at least undesirable, I don't really need to explain to the patient at all what I am intending to do, provided that I am acting in accordance with the patient's general objectives."

To go that far is to lose sight of the value of respect for autonomy. Having recognized that *fully* informed consent is an idle dream, it is necessary to decide how much information a therapist should give a patient before and during therapy. In view of the importance of respect for autonomy, a therapist should, where possible, aim to allow the patient to make an informed, rational choice about whether to have a particular therapy. This does not, in general, mean that the therapist should have to explain all the technicalities of that particular therapy, any more than informed consent to surgery requires the surgeon to explain all the details of the surgical technique. There are, as we have seen, good reasons for not, in particular circumstances, attempting a full explanation of a therapy. It could, however, mean explaining the general strategy of the therapy, what sort of commitment it is likely to require, whether there is a fee and, if so, the likely cost, and so on. As with good medical practice, the amount and detail of information given should vary according to the ability of the patient to receive and understand it. Because there is such variation between therapies, therapists, and patients, the information that must be given for consent to therapy to be sufficiently well-informed in the circumstances will vary enormously.

It might seem, therefore, that the problem of informed consent is more intractable than it is in medical practices such as surgery. From the point of view of ensuring that consent is properly informed, however, most psychotherapies have certain advantages over surgery. Psychotherapy is not a once-and-for-all irreversible procedure. Patients can get up from the couch at any time, in a way that they cannot leave the operating table. The consequences of doing so may sometimes be damaging, sometimes beneficial (see the section "Proselytizing in psychotherapy", in chapter six), but they are rarely disastrous. Furthermore, the psychotherapist, unlike the surgeon, can offer the patient a *sample* of her work and an *evolving contract*, which means that consent is gradually deepened, rather than instantly given. In an assessment interview, the psychotherapist is tacitly, or openly, saying to the patient: "This is who I am and how I operate: do you think we are likely to be able to work together?" In the private sector, the patient clearly has the option not to return, and to seek therapy elsewhere if she chooses. In state-funded psychotherapy, this freedom may be more limited, and safeguards are needed to ensure that alternative therapies and therapists are available if patients are not to feel coerced into a particular therapy with a particular therapist without proper consent.

A psychotherapy contract could perhaps be likened to other major commitments like house purchase and marriage, both of which are based on a two-phase negotiation, with a preliminary period that precedes any firm undertaking. The therapist may, if the therapy is to be prolonged, offer an initial series of, say, six sessions, after which both therapist and patient will decide if they wish to go further. It is important that regular reviews at definite intervals are built into therapies so that consent can be reconsidered in the light of the evolving process of therapy.

It is therefore very important, when considering all the reasons for not giving patients a full account of the nature of a therapy that it is proposed she have, to make sure that the reasons are at least clear to the therapist, and that they are not extended beyond their legitimate domain, thereby supporting an unwarranted or arrogant paternalism.

False memory syndrome—
deceived by memory, or memories of deceit

FALSE ACCUSATION, OR LYING FATHER?

A retired schoolmaster, a divorced man, was tending his garden one summer's day when suddenly he heard a screech of breaks outside his house. His 25-year-old daughter, with whom he thought he was on good terms, leapt out of her car, accompanied by a friend, and instantly accused him of having ruined her life by sexually abusing her when she was a child. Memories of this abuse had surfaced, she said, during the psychotherapy she had undergone in the previous year and which, ironically, he had helped to fund. He had no recollection of any such abuse, although he had bathed his daughter regularly as a child. He had been unhappily married but had waited until the children were grown up before leaving her mother. Following this incident, she broke off all contact with her father, as did her brother and sister, all of whom were convinced that he was an abuser.

Incidents such as these are not uncommon, and they place therapists in an especially difficult situation. It is certainly improper to suggest abuse when none may have occurred, but on the other hand not to search for abuse as a possible explanation for distressing symptoms might also be a dereliction of duty. Public debate about false memory has been intense and there is now an extensive literature on the subject (see, for example, British Psychological Society, 1995; Holmes, 1996; Loftus, 1993; Mollon, 1996). There is a tendency for the two sides to adopt polarized positions, and for the whole debate to become contaminated by polemic and political vituperation. In what follows, we try to step back from this and to place the current debate in its historical and scientific context.

Freud and memory

Hysterics, as every student of psychotherapy knows, suffer mainly from reminiscences—or rather from the lack of them. Based on Janet's ideas about suppression of traumatic memories, Breuer and Freud proposed the striking and daringly counter-intuitive theory that remembering and suffering were incompatible:

> Each individual hysterical symptom immediately and permanently disappeared when we had succeeded in bringing clearly to light the memory of the event by which it was provoked and in arousing its accompanying affect, and when the patient had described that event in the greatest possible detail and had put the affect into words. [Freud, 1895d, p. 6]

Note that at this stage this was simply a theory about hysteria. But from it Freud built his early "topographical" theory of a dual mind, split between an unconscious, mute, "amnesic" part, and a conscious part endowed with the power of speech. The divide was seen as the product of repression, whose purpose was to ensure that painful or threatening thoughts were "forgotten" in order to preserve the equilibrium and integrity of the psyche. The task of psychotherapy was to help overcome this divide, to "give sorrow words", originally by abreaction, later by encouragement and light pressure on the forehead, then through free association and the analysis of dreams and parapraxes, and finally through the analysis of transference, in which, Freud hypothesized, memories were enacted rather than spoken.

All this presupposed a trauma lying at the heart of neurosis. But what was the nature of this trauma? Janet's amnesic soldiers had suffered battle trauma in the Franco–Prussian war of the 1870s.

Where was the battlefield for Freud's hysterics and obsessionals? It was, of course, the family, especially perhaps the claustrophobic middle-class Jewish family life of fin-de-siècle Vienna from which most of Freud's early patients came. Hence the famous "seduction hypothesis". Hysteria stemmed from "pre-sexual sexual shock" (Freud, 1896c) during the "first period of childhood" when "mnemic residues are not translated into verbal images".

Here we see the blurring of the boundary between theory and observation which has made psychoanalysis so attractive, especially to those of a speculative turn of mind, but it also represents its Achilles heel. The "seduction hypothesis" was elegant and powerful and suggested a clear therapeutic goal. But its empirical basis was flimsy. For a start, most of the accounts of childhood seduction proposed by Freud were not directly reported or remembered but inferred—indeed, the very nature of his hypothesis meant that this had to be so. Freud would read evidence of sexuality into his patients' hysterical postures, hallucinatory sensations, and mental imagery and then powerfully suggest to them that these were manifestations of repressed memories of seduction (Schimek, 1985). If the patient denied his suggestions, he would threaten her:

> She is now in the throes of the most vehement resistance. . . . I have threatened to send her away and in the process convinced myself that she has already gained a good deal of certainty which she is reluctant to acknowledge. [Freud, 1887–1904. pp. 220–221]

A second point of contradiction is that in many of the cases described in *Studies in Hysteria*, the "seduction" occurs not in infancy as the theory demands, but in childhood or early adolescence, and usually the facts themselves—if not their emotional import—are recalled without much difficulty by the sufferer. Already Freud (1896c) is suggesting that it is not so much the anamnesis itself as the significance, connections, and affective response to the trauma that are problematic. "Katerina", for example, whom Freud "analysed" in a single session while on a walking trip in the mountains, clearly recalled her "uncle" (actually it was her father) climbing into her bed and pressing his body against her when she was 14. Freud's intervention was to connect this memory not with infantile trauma, but with the presenting feelings of giddiness and nausea brought on by her witnessing this same "uncle" in a sexually compromising situation with her cousin (Sabbadini, 1992).

As is well known, by 1897 Freud was beginning to have doubts about the "seduction hypothesis", although it was to be another seven years before he publicly repudiated it. His doubts were based on four basic difficulties. First, he found, contrary to his assertion in *Studies in Hysteria*, that most patients confronted with the "facts" of their seduction did not automatically get better. It seemed that simply putting trauma into words—always assuming that the trauma had occurred in the first place—did not in itself produce cure. Second, he could not believe that infantile seduction could be so widespread as the hypothesis required—have *all* neurotics' fathers abused them in infancy? Third, he began to wonder if patient's "memories" were not at least in part created by his own suggestions. Finally, he began to question the capacity of the infantile mind to distinguish clearly between actual events and phantasies (Blass & Simon, 1994).

Phantasy, of course, provided the starting point for his next period of intense theorizing and forms the kernel of what we now see as psychoanalysis proper, as opposed to this "pre-psychoanalytic" phase. Through the notion of "screen memories", Freud hypothesized that both current preoccupations and infantile phantasies could be disguised and "re-presented" to consciousness as though they were actual occurrences (Freud, 1899a). He now decided that the supposed seductions at the hands of parents and other adults contained within them the subject's *own* infantile erotic longings and phantasies. Note that this does not eliminate the possibility of real trauma in the origin of neurosis. The undoubted traumatic seductions of late childhood and early adolescence would then derive their force from the infantile phantasies that they re-evoke—as Neville Symington puts it, "reality confirms the phantasy" (personal communication, 1985).

By his repudiation of the "seduction hypothesis", Freud has of course been accused of "betrayal", contributing to the widespread social and medical denial of the reality that adults *do* sexually abuse young children and to the likelihood that this significantly contributes to psychological illness in later life. Freud clearly continued to be troubled by this issue throughout his career, and in "Constructions in Analysis", one of his last papers, he returned to the subject (Freud, 1937d). Here there is a significant shift compared with his early ideas. He clearly asserts that it is not so much the *facts* that are forgotten, but the associated feelings:

There are hints of repetitions of the *affects* belonging to the repressed material to be found in actions performed by the patient
. . . some fairly important, some trivial, both inside and outside
the analytic situation. [Freud, 1937d, p. 258; italics added]

The "repressed material"—that which is "forgotten"—manifests itself
in inappropriate affective responses.

NOT FACTS, BUT FEELINGS, ARE FORGOTTEN

For example, a teacher whose beloved father had died three years
earlier had rather precipitately returned to her home town to take
up a job as a deputy-head. She immediately found herself at log-
gerheads with the headmaster, whom she saw as a petty-minded
sycophant more interested in his own career and fulfilling the
requirements of the educational authorities than in the welfare of
the children. This conflict precipitated a major depression in
which she felt she had ruined everything and failed utterly. In
therapy, she immediately formed a rather idealized relationship
with her older male therapist. When asked to compare the headmaster with her father (also a teacher), she said forcibly "but they
couldn't be more different if they tried!". It was only when she
realized that her fury with this man was that he was not her
father, whom she had unconsciously hoped to retrieve through
her job move, that she began to understand her feelings of frustration and misery.

What was "forgotten" were not the facts of the case—she was well
aware of her deep "oedipal" love for her father and her sadness at his
death. She was unconscious not so much of the facts, but of the
emotional context in which they arose—the connections between past
and present—and the way in which "unprocessed" affects—her feelings of grief, anger, disappointment, longing for intimacy with a lost
loved one—were motivating her actions, influencing her perceptions,
and so leading to a transference onto her new headmaster.

Freud gives the example of offering a "construction" to a patient:

"Up to your nth year you regarded yourself as the sole and
unlimited possessor of your mother; then came another baby
and brought you grave disillusionment. Your mother left you
for some time, and even after her reappearance she was never

devoted to you exclusively. Your feelings towards your mother became ambivalent, your father gained a new importance for you . . ." and so on. [Freud, 1937d, p. 261]

Here, again, what is being provided is not a hitherto repressed memory, but a *context* in which a set of difficult feelings—disappointment, rivalry, ambivalence, and so on—can be understood. The patient has not forgotten the facts of life itself (except perhaps in the extreme case of fugue states and severe dissociation) but has lost touch with the feelings associated with the facts, and the web of meanings they entail.

Freud goes on to discuss the question of validation: how do we know whether the "constructions" offered to the patient are true or not? His answer comes from what he somewhat disingenuously describes as "indirect forms of confirmation which are in every respect trustworthy". He claims that when the patient responds by saying "'I didn't ever think of that' . . . This can be translated without hesitation into 'Yes, you are right this time—about my *unconscious*'" (p. 268; italics in original). But when patients respond in this way, it usually seems to mean that the therapist has got it wrong in some way, and that the patient is too polite to say so (a point that is often germane to their difficulties): either the "construction" is way off beam or, even if correct, it is a premature interpretation. At this point, the relationship between therapist and patient becomes asymmetrical: the therapist is imposing something, rather than working collaboratively.

This suspicion is rather confirmed by an extraordinary passage that Freud uses to back up his assertion about "indirect confirmation". He describes how a colleague brought his wife for a consultation—admittedly one that was, in Freud's phrase, "extra-analytic"—because she "refused on all sort of pretexts to have sexual relations with him" (p. 265). Freud's role was to give her a dressing down, which he duly did, explaining how she was endangering their marriage and so forth, whereupon the husband exclaimed: "That Englishman you diagnosed as suffering from a cerebral tumour has died too". Freud adduces the extraneous "too" as evidence of an "indirect confirmation" from the husband's unconscious which is, as it were, saying to his wife "he was right in that case also!", via this fragment of linguistic slippage. But surely what is happening here is that husband and therapist are lined up to bully the wife into submission, and could not the same process occur when a patient is asked to swallow one of the therapist's "constructions"?

Current "post-psychoanalytic" thought emphasizes the power relationship between analyst and patient. Livingston Smith (1991) suggests that the "seduction hypothesis" was a projection into the past of the *current* therapist–patient relationship (the "penetrating" interpretations, the resistant but helpless patient, etc.). For many feminist writers, Freud's disavowal of infantile seduction and insistence that these "memories" originated in the patient's phantasies equally proves that he was abusing his authority to deny the reality of childhood abuse. Both of these perspectives concede that "memory" is potentially unreliable, and that what appears to be "remembered" has to be evaluated in a much wider context, especially that of the therapeutic relationship. In *Macbeth*, Macduff is speechless when he first hears that his wife and three children have been murdered. Malcolm gently urges him to "give sorrow words". For Shakespeare, "the grief that cannot speak/whispers the o'er-fraught heart, and bids it break". Repression is interpersonal: Macduff has not repressed the reality of the loss (he can "whisper" it to himself); if only he can "speak" it to his friends, his risk of heartbreak is lessened.

Freud ends his paper with two main points. The first seems to be the concession that, in the last analysis, one can never be sure if a "construction" is true, but that

> If the analysis is carried out correctly, we produce in him an assured conviction of the truth of the construction *which achieves the same therapeutic result as a recaptured memory.* [Freud, 1937d, p. 266; italics added]

For someone who had fought all his life to differentiate psychoanalysis from "suggestion", this seems to be an extraordinary conclusion, since he seems to be saying, just as do Spence (1982) and Schafer (1983) half a century later, that so long as the patient gets better it does not matter whether or not the "construction" is historically correct.

Freud then moves from a discussion of "ultra-clear" memories that turn out to be false, to the speculation that psychotic delusions may constitute attempts at "reconstruction", containing within them fragments of historical events. Both of these points are relevant to our discussion. First, the clarity of memories, as opposed to the hazy quality of dreams and phantasy, may well be the method by which we decide on their veracity; thus an "ultra-clear" phantasy can easily, by perceptual "mis-attribution", be labelled as a memory (a point originally made in the eighteenth century by Berkeley). Second, while Freud argues that hallucinations may contain fragments of reality (as they undoubtedly do), it is equally possible—indeed, it is inherent in their definition—that fragments of hallucination may be misinterpreted as reality.

Memory and contemporary psychoanalytic psychotherapy

A striking feature of contemporary psychoanalytic psychotherapy is the way in which "repression"—for Freud, such a central concept—has imperceptibly faded into the background (Bateman & Holmes, 1995). This follows from an equally radical shift in the way in which the unconscious is understood. For Freud, the unconscious and repression were virtually synonymous: that which we cannot remember is always a result of an active process of forgetting. The advent of object relations meant that the inner world is no longer viewed as a storehouse of repressed drives and memories, but in terms of a *representational* world in which internal objects are formed out of a complex blend of phantasy and memories of actual experience.

In addition, contemporary views of the unconscious have changed in response to a widened psychotherapeutic culture that is open to non-analytic findings and ideas. These include the findings of cognitive science, changing clinical experience, and as a manifestation of shifting cultural perspectives.

Cognitive science and contemporary psychoanalytic psychotherapy. The first notion that has to be questioned in the light of cognitive science is that of "infantile amnesia" (Lindsay & Read, 1994). Since amnesia for the first two years of life is virtually universal, rather than invoking "primary repression", it seems more parsimonious to assume that there is a neurological/maturational basis for such lack of memory, and that the advent of language around 2 years is linked in some way with the beginnings of what Tulving (1985) calls "episodic memory"—the ability to recall specific events and situations. That is not to say that the experiences of the first two years of life have no effects, or are not in some way "layed down" in the nervous system. Quite the contrary: Tulving differentiates the episodic memory system from what he calls "semantic" and "procedural" memory. Semantic memory refers to the "grammar" of our lives: the rules of relationships that are just as ingrained as are actual happenings, which Byng-Hall (1995), after Schank (1982), calls "event-scripts". Procedural memory would be akin to Segal's (1991) "memory in the body", the somatic sensations of intimacy, rejection, satiation, frustration, and so on that form a psychophysiological substrate to the sense of self (what we and the world "feels" like) and is presumably related to parental handling in the early months of life.

A second radical break with Freudian metapsychology follows from the study of unconscious perception (Bornstein, 1993). Freud saw perception and consciousness as inseparable (the "system Pcpt.-Cs."). For him, perceptions were pristine: only memories were subject to repression. Thus, to put it schematically, a perception might evoke memories of infantile desire which would then be repressed and therefore removed from consciousness and so manifest themselves via neurotic symptoms. Repression, in this model, is always operating on the past, never the present. But we now know that perception itself is linked to the current state of the organism. There is a feedback loop between memory and perception itself. We literally do turn a blind eye to disturbing percepts, in the sense that they do not necessarily register with consciousness even though they can be shown to affect subsequent performance and, even more intriguingly, there is evidence that brain-damaged individuals who cannot consciously "see" stimuli are in fact influenced by them (via so-called "blindsight": Bornstein, 1993). We are unconsciously aware of far more than we consciously "know". If the aim of psychotherapy is still that of increasing the field of awareness ("where id was, there ego shall be"), this no longer simply means releasing imprisoned memories from the past, but, rather, widening the perceptual field in the present.

A second shift away from the classical psychoanalytic position concerns the nature of defence, of which repression is the prototypical example. For Freud, defence mechanisms were just that—*mechanisms* by which painful or unacceptable thoughts were kept from consciousness. We now conceive a much more fluid relationship between consciousness and the rest of the mind. We may be completely unaware or dimly aware or may consciously suppress painful feelings and memories; or, at times of stress and depression, we may feel overwhelmed by them.

THE RETURN OF THE REPRESSED

A depressed man in his 40s "knew" that his father had been alcoholic and had died when he was 11, that his brother had died in a road accident a year later, and that his mother had had a depressive breakdown soon afterwards, but he never talked about these events to anyone, even, as he put it "to myself". It was only when he began to be overwhelmed with feelings of sadness and futility around the time that his son reached the age of 11, and he was himself slightly injured in a minor road accident, that he sought help. In the setting of therapy, vivid images from the past came flooding back—the mixture of sympathy and disgust he experienced when he helped his father to walk to the off-licence (which he then linked for the first time with his chosen career as a nurse), and the sexual abuse he had undergone when, desperate for affection and security, he was "looked after" by an "uncle" while his mother was in hospital (which he could then begin to link with his exaggeratedly "macho" approach to life and relationships with women).

In summary, the recovery of memory in therapy may take one of three forms. First, the patient may be helped to get in touch with current thoughts and phantasies of which she is dimly aware but has failed to attend to, or to realize how much she may be influencing day-to-day moods and behaviour. Second, there may be the emergence of genuinely repressed traumatic memories, as in classical psychoanalysis. Third, and most contentiously, there are putative memories which may be inherently unrecoverable in "semantic" form—if they date to a time before the age of 2—but which may be inferred from the patient's history, collateral evidence, and behaviour in relation to the therapist.

In the light of this discussion, we can now briefly comment on the controversy surrounding recovered memories and the so-called false memory syndrome. It seems that many counsellors and therapists base their work around Freud's pre-1897 model of hysteria: symptoms equal repression equals abuse, therefore therapy equals remembering equals recovery. It as though the whole subsequent history and findings of psychoanalysis and cognitive psychology had not happened (Weiskrantz, 1995). But there is still truth in these original ideas, especially in relation to childhood abuse. Memories are often kept out of awareness and, when they do surface, threaten to overwhelm the sufferer, who often develops symptoms that in the nineteenth century might have been labelled as "hysteria"—feelings of panic, nausea, dizziness, sexual difficulties, and so on. The "recovery" of memories often arises out of a contemporaneous trigger, such as a relationship difficulty or a child reaching the age that the sufferer was when she was abused. These people appear to have been deprived of the soothing and comfort associated with secure attachment. Many turn to various forms of surrogate soothing: self-harm, alcohol and drugs, or eating disorders. Self-harm soothes presumably because it distracts from mental pain, a dissociative technique that many "discovered" as a way of enduring the abuse. Chaotic relationships, alcohol and substance abuse, or bulimia also fulfil a threefold function of distraction, possible endogenous opiate release, and the evoking of protective behaviour in carers (De Zuluetta, 1993).

What epidemiological evidence there is suggests that total amnesia for trauma and abuse is rare, although, as already mentioned, amnesia for events before the age of 2 years is almost universal. In one study of women who were known to have been abused in childhood, only 20 per cent had no recollection of it (Lindsay & Read, 1994). Much more common are patterns of unassimilated memory as described above: facts are recalled but not feelings, or the individual develops trance-like states in which past and present are confused.

There is also prima facie evidence that "false memories" are possible, even if their incidence may be fairly low. It is well known that the past takes on a depressive colouring in depressive illness, and that apparent trauma is often forgotten or denied when the subject recovers. Similarly, depressed people regress to a paranoid–schizoid state in which there is an urgent need to blame and attack, which may resolve when they feel better. There is also good evidence that memories can be "created" by suggestion. Mis-recall is enhanced in those ways that would be particularly likely to occur in an intense therapeutic relationship: when the one who suggests is in a position of authority; when the time gap between the event and the suggestion is great; when the suggestions are frequently repeated; when they are plausible; and when initially the subject is merely asked to give a yes/no answer—this then leading to circumstantial elaboration. Individuals vary in their suggestibility, and those who are "field-dependent" are most likely to mis-recall—ironically, they are also those who are most likely to have been abused.

At its worst, "false memory" can arise out of simple errors of logic. *Post hoc, propter hoc* bedevils discussion of causality in psychotherapy generally. Even if the simple recovery of memories did lead to cure—and there is very little evidence that it does—that would not in itself prove that forgetting of trauma is necessarily pathogenic. Childhood trauma and abuse undoubtedly comprise significant vulnerability factors for adult psychiatric disorder, but they are not in themselves causative (Mullen, Romans-Clarkson, Walton, & Herbison, 1993). We need to know much more about the intervening variables, of which "memory", in the sense of how the world is and was construed, is one of the most significant. A second simple error of logic is that of the "undistributed middle". Thus the argument, "bulimic women have been sexually abused in childhood, you are bulimic, therefore you must have been sexually abused in childhood (even if you have no recall)", is logically unsound—although apparently widely believed by therapists (Poole, Lindsay, Memon, & Bull, 1995).

We conclude this section with another example illustrating how the *context* in which abuse is discussed may have a determining effect on whether it is "remembered" or "forgotten".

REPRESSION WITHIN THERAPY

A teacher in her 30s suffered from bouts of crippling depression. She got on very badly with her father and found him repellent for reasons that she could not quite understand. It emerged that her mother had suffered from postnatal depression and had spent several months in hospital when the patient was 3 years old. The patient had been looked after by her father at that time, her grandparents having died. After several weeks of discussion around this topic, the therapist gently speculated about whether some kind of abuse might have occurred then, which would perhaps explain her subsequent feelings of revulsion. The patient took this suggestion up vigorously, became convinced of its truth, and cut off all relations with her parents. The therapist, feeling guilty that he might have implanted this idea in the patient's mind for which there was no objective evidence, was at pains to remind her that it was only speculation. His guilt was enhanced when he received a letter from the patient's mother accusing him of poisoning the mother–daughter relationship. The topic then disappeared from therapy for some time. Much later, the patient told the therapist that her mother had confirmed the abuse, but she (the patient) had decided not to bring it up in therapy any more, since the therapist clearly was uncomfortable with the topic!

Sexual exploitation in therapy

There is a popular, though not entirely fair, image of male psycho-therapists as powerful figures who, Svengali-like, seduce their helpless female patients. The sexual exploitation of patients by thera-pists is an obvious topic of ethical concern, even though psychiatrists and other therapists report that, rather than patients being seduced by therapists, what is much more common is that patients pursue *them* for sexual contact. Before considering the ethics of therapist–patient sex, we should ask how widespread such practice is, for if it were really only an isolated occurrence, discussion of it would, for many, be of merely academic interest. In a paper in the *American Journal of Psychiatry*, Gartrell and her colleagues (1986) published the results of a survey into sexual relationships between psychiatrists and patients in the United States. Although their survey was by no means exhaustive, its results were similar to an earlier study of psy-chologists (Holyroyd & Brodsky, 1977). The extent of sexual contacts is shown by this summary of their findings:

> In a nationwide survey of U.S. psychiatrists, 7.1% (1057) of the male and 3.1% (257) of the female respondents acknowledged sexual contact with their own patients. Eighty-eight per cent of the sexual contacts occurred between male psychiatrists and fe-male patients. All offenders who had been involved with more than one patient were male. [Gartrell et al., 1986]

Subsequent surveys have confirmed that sexual exploitation of patients is a regular, if relatively infrequent, occurrence in therapy. It would thus appear that sexual contact between therapist and patient, although by no means ubiquitous, is more than just an isolated occur-rence that could safely be ignored, especially as these admitted sexual liaisons are likely to be an underestimate, in virtue of the shame of admitting that one has engaged in a strongly disapproved of activity.

It is almost universally thought to be quite wrong for a therapist and patient to develop a sexual relationship during therapy, in or out of the consulting room, But what *is* wrong with it, provided that both parties consent, and what, if anything, should be done to prevent it?

One strong objection to therapists having sexual relationships with their patients is that it is exploitative. Exploitation is the taking advantage of an imbalance in power to further the exploiter's own interests at the expense of the party with less power. So defined, all exploitation is wrong, since it is inconsistent with respect for individual autonomy. But is it exploitative for a therapist to enter into a sexual relationship with a patient?

With many professional relationships, such as those between bank managers or architects and their clients, and including that between therapist and patient, there is an obvious sense in which a sexual relationship could be exploitative. This is where the professional either directly or indirectly requires sexual favours in return for professional services. By relying on professional help, one puts oneself, to a certain extent, at the mercy of the professional. This creates an imbalance of power, which the professional should not exploit for her own advantage at the expense of her client.

There is, however, no *principled* reason why architect and client should not freely enter into a sexual relationship. Nor is there any principled objection to having an affair or lasting relationship with one's bank manager. It might, however, be proper under these circumstances for the manager to hand her customer/lover's account over to a colleague, in order to ensure that no unwarranted bias entered into professional transactions, and that the bank was seen to be concerned that this did not happen.

Although it is difficult to estimate the precise harm that therapist–patient sex causes, Gartrell's study revealed that an overwhelming majority of psychiatrists believe that sexual contact between therapist and patient is always inappropriate, usually or always harmful, and in many cases equivalent to rape. Rape is a serious criminal offence, and a therapist, like anyone else found guilty of rape, should suffer a severe legal penalty. But most therapist–patient sex certainly falls short of rape. Should such contact be a criminal offence? If not, should it be controlled, and if so how? An opponent of control might, on anti-paternalistic grounds, argue in the following way.

The mere fact that an activity is thought to be harmful to those who choose to engage in it is not generally thought to be a sufficient reason for banning it. Otherwise, cigarette smoking, high-cholesterol foods, and low-exercise, stressful lifestyles might all be banned. Such a ban would constitute an excessive invasion of individual liberty. Provided that a psychotherapy patient is not below the legal age of consent and is not, by way of mental disorder, incapable of making a competent choice, to ban therapist–patient sex would, like banning high-cholesterol foods, constitute a violation of respect for the autonomy of patient and therapist alike. If a patient freely consents to a sexual relationship with a therapist, and especially if the patient initiates the relationship, it would be wrong for an outside agency to meddle in their private affairs.

The force of this argument is that, unless one is prepared to accept a very strong authoritarianism, the case for banning therapist–patient sexual contact should not rest solely on the claim that such contact is likely to harm therapist or patient. People are not normally banned from engaging in risky or harmful behaviour, provided that nobody else is directly harmed by it and they have freely chosen their course of action. But we should not conclude from this that therapist–patient sex ought to be permitted, for there may be other grounds for seeking its prohibition.

First, the therapeutic relationship, by virtue of the phenomena of transference and countertransference, produces special circumstances that are likely both to arouse erotic feelings and to undermine the patient's, and possibly the therapist's, capacity to make a sound judgement about the desirability of sexual contact (see Gabbard, 1996). There is almost invariably a strong connection between sexual exploitation in therapy and patients who have been sexually abused as children. Indeed, in its most heinous form, sexually abusive therapists will justify sleeping with their patients on the grounds that a "healing" sexual experience is needed to counteract the damaging effects of childhood sexual abuse!

The feelings that are generated in therapy may be very powerful and are, especially in analytic therapies, therapeutic provided that they are observed and understood but *not* acted on. If they are acted on *within* therapy they almost inevitably destroy the therapeutic space which allows feelings to be expressed and explored safely, and these feelings are most unlikely to be appropriate in the real world *outside* therapy. Let us recall Freud's own statement about transference, which indicates why this might be so:

> If someone's need for love is not entirely satisfied by reality he is bound to approach every new person he meets with libidinal anticipatory ideas—and it is highly probable that both portions of his libido, the portion that is capable of becoming conscious as well as the unconscious one, have a share in forming that attitude. . . . It is a perfectly normal and intelligible thing that this should be directed to the figure of the doctor. [Freud, 1912b]

Acting directly on feelings generated within therapy is not only dangerous, but is most likely to be the product of irrational desires and fantasies. In view of this, we should *not* regard sexual encounters within individual therapy as the product of autonomous choices made by the participants. When Oedipus killed his father and married his mother, his actions were heteronomous since founded on crucially false beliefs. It would not have been inconsistent with respect for Oedipus's autonomy for someone who knew the identity of his parents to prevent him from doing what he did. This is quite different from a case where someone acts in full awareness of what she is doing. Although the aim of therapy is greater emotional autonomy, including coming to terms with one's emotions as they really are, therapy itself can be intoxicating. From the point of view of respect for individual autonomy, for a therapist to allow a sexual encounter to develop is analogous to getting someone drunk and then seducing her.

Related to this point is the fear that if therapist–patient sex *were* permitted, this could put pressure on a patient or a therapist to respond to the inappropriate sexual overtures of the other, and thus undermine the therapy. The situation is made even more difficult by the fact that, as we have argued, caring and loving are an important part of psychotherapy, and physical contact between patient and therapist may be a legitimate part of this. Martin Lakin points out that

> Therapists often make a distinction between erotic and nonerotic physical contact. Sometimes, and with some patients, touching is seen as a way—often the only apparent way—of establishing important emotional communication. Although touching may arouse fears of invasive contact or sexual exploitation that can reach panic levels, it may also be important for calming a panic state in the person, and for many experiencing depression—for

example grieving individuals—touching is a way to express reassurance and solace. [Lakin, 1988]

It is most important that there be clear boundaries between erotic and non-erotic loving, between erotic and non-erotic physical contact. If, say, a patient *does* make overtures to a therapist, the responsible therapist's rejection of the advances will be made easier, less indicative of rejection, if there is a strict rule: "Therapist–patient sexual relationships are absolutely forbidden."

This brings us to another reason for thinking that there should be restrictions on therapist–patient sex. Sexual contact in therapy is most unlikely to be therapeutically beneficial. The sequel to Gartrell's study revealed that less than 2 per cent of the respondents thought that therapist–patient sex "could be appropriate for the enhancement of the patient's self-esteem, as a corrective emotional experience for the patient, to shorten a grief reaction, or to convert a patient from one sexual orientation to another" (Gartrell et al., 1988). There is evidence that therapist–patient sex actually undermines the goals of therapy. If this is correct, then therapists who have sex with their patients may be guilty, wittingly or not, of misleading their patients. They have offered them one thing, on the basis of which the patient agrees to enter into the relationship; but what the patient receives is something that is not only different from what was offered, but is also likely to defeat the goals for which the offer was accepted in the first place.

There will undoubtedly be the occasional case where "spontaneous" therapist–patient sex does not seriously undermine therapy, and takes place with the genuine full consent of both parties. But because such cases are likely to be rare and difficult to predict in advance, and because the temptations for sexual contact in therapy are high, there is a good case for banning it.

It is not clear, however, except in the case of rape, that therapist–patient sex should be a crime: it is, at most, a civil wrong. Therapists who allow sexual relationships to develop with patients are not necessarily criminals or villains, but they certainly lack the heightened sense of moral responsibility that we have argued is an essential characteristic of a good therapist. They are also bad therapists, in that they are caught up in the enactment of a phantasy rather than being able to stand back from their countertransference feelings and see them for what they are.

We believe that therapist–patient sex should be banned from within psychotherapy. But how should this be effected? Because of the civil liberties arguments mentioned above, we do not believe that direct legal proscription would be desirable. The most effective alternative would be for the ban to be enforced by a psychotherapy *profession*, which, via the various registers (the most extensive of which is that of the UKCP: see chapter ten), has the power, via the training organization to which the offending therapist belongs, to determine who should and should not be an accredited psychotherapist. We consider this further in chapters nine and ten.

The only likely exception to the ban might be those so-called therapies based around sexual surrogacy, which make it clear in advance to their patients that they rely on therapist–patient sex, but these are better thought of as benign forms of prostitution rather than falling within any acceptable definition of psychotherapy. (In this connection, Freud is said to have had a working arrangement with certain prostitutes in Vienna to whom he would "refer" his impotent clients once their analysis had reached a suitable stage! The fact that the focus of psychotherapy has now shifted from male impotence to female sexual abuse is a mark of the cultural resonance of therapy.)

There is, however, one difficult residual problem. What happens if therapist and patient genuinely fall in love in the course of treatment and want to form a sexual relationship beyond the therapy? Although there are no easy answers, this is the sort of problem that psychotherapists should address.

A therapist who finds herself falling in love with a patient should almost certainly refer the patient to another therapist as soon as possible. Would it be morally permissible for a therapist to start a sexual relationship with an ex-patient once therapy has stopped, or once the patient has been referred to another therapist? There is clearly less reason for proposing a ban on sex with ex-patients than on sex during therapy. However, some of the problems associated with therapist–patient sex during therapy remain. For example, transference-based feelings are unlikely suddenly to cease when formal therapy comes to an end. Moreover, a patient may temporarily leave therapy only to return.

Good practice would certainly require a cooling-off period after therapist and patient had stopped seeing each other professionally. But it would, perhaps, be undesirable for a psychotherapy profession to attempt to impose a ban on sexual relationships between therapists and ex-patients. In one case, a psychiatrist was struck off the medical register for having a sexual relationship with a patient whom he had referred to another therapist (because he realized he was falling in love with her), and whom he subsequently married; this seems unduly harsh. However, as therapists should be very wary of establishing sexual relationships with ex-patients, because of the transference effect, good practice would require a cooling-off period of perhaps six months or a year. This could be recommended, though perhaps not enforced, by the UKCP via the training organizations.

Financial exploitation in therapy: paying too much for too long

One of the most frequently expressed worries about private analytic psychotherapy, felt even by those who recognize its benefits, is the possibility of financial exploitation in interminable therapy. This is a particular problem for analytic psychotherapy because of its indeterminate goals and indefinite length. Most therapies create a temporary dependency, but with a view to creating long-term enhanced autonomy. It may even be the case that some patients *need* indefinite, perhaps lifelong, therapeutic dependency to stave off more serious mental incapacity, and so retain a modicum of autonomy. But within the private sector, where fees are the subject of private negotiation between patient and therapist, there is a risk that a patient will be paying high fees over a long period without the therapy actually getting anywhere. It is possible for unscrupulous therapists to maintain this arrangement by ensuring that their patients remain permanently dependent upon them. This then becomes a form of exploitation, since the therapist uses a position of relative power to take advantage of the patient.

A libertarian such as Szasz would argue that the principle of *caveat emptor!* [let the buyer beware!] should govern private psychotherapy contracts, and that the only regulation should be to prevent fraud, where the seller sells under false pretences by giving false or misleading information to the customer. Any further restriction would be a paternalistic interference with liberty, which failed to respect the individual autonomy of consumers.

We believe that the nature of the therapeutic relationship places psychotherapy in a very different position from, say, the sale of consumer durables. As we have argued, therapy often generates a dependency of patient on therapist, which in the long run can help the patient to become more independent and autonomous. The special risks associated with this mean that patients do need protection against financial exploitation.

The free market is, in many ways, efficient and equitable, but there are situations where it notoriously fails. It fails, for example, to secure justice for those suffering from a bargaining disadvantage. Such is the position of psychotherapy patients, for two reasons: first, as Foster (1971) pointed out, those seeking psychotherapy are likely to include "the weak, the insecure, the lonely, the inadequate and the depressed", second, therapy itself creates its own temporary dependency. In these respects, the relationship between therapist and patient is different from that between television seller and purchaser.

A second situation where a free market is not efficient and equitable is where information costs for the consumer are high. If there are over 300 kinds of therapy, and if, in addition, every therapist is a unique commodity, the information costs to the consumer of finding out which therapy or therapist is most appropriate are enormous. Under these circumstances, a completely free market is neither an efficient nor an equitable mechanism for the distribution of psychotherapy.

At present, with no professional organization for psychotherapy, it is possible for therapists to charge whatever they can persuade their patients to pay, and to continue receiving money from patients for a long period, irrespective of whether they are doing them any good. An effective way to combat the problem of overcharging would be for the profession to establish an agreed scale of fees for psychotherapy, as is common practice in certain other professions.

We do not believe that it is realistic to propose free publicly funded analytic psychotherapy for everyone who needs or demands it, for reasons given in chapter four: it would be too expensive and is, anyway, not suitable for everyone. But we do think that steps should be taken to make analytic psychotherapy more widely available to the less well-off. One way of doing this would be for the professional scale of fees to be related to ability to pay, so that the better-off would effectively subsidize the worse-off. Indeed, schemes like this do already exist in the private sector. Another possibility might be the establishment of a psychotherapeutic equivalent of the legal aid fund, which provides free or subsidized legal representation for those whose income is below a certain level.

The problem of interminable therapy is more interesting and more difficult to resolve than that of overcharging, particularly because of the problem of who is to say whether the continuation of therapy is necessary or beneficial for the patient. A libertarian would say that this is purely a matter for patient and therapist to decide— just as with any other professional contractual relationship. However, as we have stressed, a psychotherapy patient is likely to be in a weak bargaining position and may well rely on guidance from the therapist to decide whether or not to continue in therapy. Moreover, a therapist may have a direct financial incentive to continue a lucrative therapeutic relationship, even if it is doing the patient no good.

A further complication is that a therapist may herself become dependent on a particular therapeutic relationship—not purely financially, but also emotionally. For example, the therapist may in good faith have difficulty in confronting the imperfections in her own life and world and may perpetuate her therapeutic relationships as a refuge from those imperfections. It is clearly unethical for a therapist to persuade a patient to stay in therapy, or not to make arrangements for her to leave therapy, in order to gratify her own unconscious needs.

Again, it may be clear what good practice would be, but less clear what, beyond appeal to therapists' consciences and good sense, should be done to prevent abuse. The problem could be somewhat alleviated if it were made a requirement that before taking on a patient a therapist should discuss with her what the objectives of the proposed therapy are, how long the therapy is likely to last, what the chances of success are, and so on. The need for a good assessment interview carried out by a practitioner who is conversant with the various forms of psychotherapy and is capable of discussing with potential patients which of these is most likely to benefit them is relevant here. Many therapists recognize these points. To make them a more formal requirement would have the virtue of making the patient's initial decision to enter therapy better informed.

There are, however, two serious objections to making such a procedure mandatory. First, at the outset of therapy it is often difficult to predict how the therapy will turn out, how long it will last, and what problems will be revealed during it. This could be partly overcome by expecting the initial statement by the therapist to incorporate these uncertainties, and by developing the idea of an evolving contract with built-in renegotiation points, which we have already mentioned. The aim would not be to preclude new developments within the therapy, but simply to put the patient in a better position to decide whether she wants to make a commitment to therapy, and to a temporary dependency on the therapist.

The second objection is, unfortunately, more difficult to meet. An attempt to communicate all the uncertainties associated with therapy, and to explain in advance how the therapy is expected to work, runs the danger of imposing a view of therapy, and therefore, rather than enhancing autonomy, undermining it. This is particularly a problem for transference-based therapies where the *patient's* (as opposed to the therapist's) expectations, assumptions, and fantasies about therapy are a vital starting point for exploration. This is really a special case of the problem of informed consent. In some circumstances, it may be that the more the therapist, as it were, shows her hand, the less likely it is that the patient will be able to show hers. As discussed in chapter six, in transference-based therapies a balance has to be struck between openness and therapeutic reticence.

We do not, therefore, think it reasonable to require therapists to give their patients more than an outline of the principles of the therapy at the outset. However, it is important that therapists do not deceive their patients into expecting one sort of treatment when they are likely to receive another.

To help overcome the problem of interminable, inefficacious therapy, we also suggest that it should be a requirement of long-term therapy that after each given period of, say, six months, the progress of the therapy should be reviewed and, if appropriate, the objectives altered in the light of developments during that time. This would, of course, be open to abuse by a genuinely unscrupulous therapist, who might be quite capable of using the review in a way that leads to agreement to further treatment, even when this is not required. However, having pointed out the vulnerabilities of patients, one should not underestimate the capacity of a patient who has had therapy for several months to be able to form a rational assessment of whether or not it is doing any good. Requiring regular reviews of long-term therapy would provide a useful, though by no means foolproof, way of evaluating progress.

A central theme of all these ethical problems that occur within psychotherapy is that respect for the autonomy of an individual is not straightforward. Respecting someone's autonomy seems to require that she be allowed to do what she chooses. However, people may, unless restricted, choose to act in ways that subvert their own autonomy. The dilemmas discussed in this chapter arise out of the particular responsibilities towards the patient that a therapeutic relationship creates in a therapist. In the next chapter, we discuss problems that arise out of the fact that therapists, although responsible to their patients, also remain members of society, with social responsibilities.

CHAPTER EIGHT

Psychotherapists:
servants of two masters?

In the previous two chapters, we focused on the responsibility that therapists assume for their patients. Part of this seems to require therapists, in a sense, to be the champions and advocates of their patients. Many of the moral dilemmas faced by therapists arise out of the ambiguities entailed in trying to respect patients' autonomy. In this chapter, we discuss another range of problems, related to the fact that therapists, like everyone else, remain citizens of a society—and, however much they might wish otherwise, that society cannot be ignored. There may be circumstances where the broader society's interests may conflict with the interests of a patient. There are also occasions where the patient's interests may conflict with another individual, a "third party". How should these conflicts be resolved?

The main libertarian worry about the state's involvement in the care and treatment of the mentally distressed or disturbed is, we argued in chapter five, the fear that large-scale state-organized mental health services will inevitably be used as an oppressive tool of social control, undermining the fundamental liberty of social dissenters to enact their dissent. Nowhere is this thought to be more a cause for concern than in the compulsory detention and treatment of the mentally ill. We argued in chapter five that such a worry, if directed against psychotherapy, *is* misplaced. Unlike drug treatments, most psychotherapy cannot be "administered" against the will of its patients, and the nature of psychotherapeutic explorations makes them especially likely to be autonomy-enhancing.

Although it may be impossible literally to force someone to undergo psychotherapy, there may, however, be situations where the main reason for offering a patient psychotherapy is not to serve the *patient's* best interests, but to promote the goals of society, to solve a social problem. A group of people whose treatment gives legitimate cause for concern are patients already within the custody or control of state authorities, or threatened with this if they do not agree to have therapy. The most obvious cases concern the use of psychotherapy with prison inmates, and its use with minors subject to or threatened with compulsory care orders. We consider these cases in turn.

Psychotherapy in the prison context

In Patuxent Penitentiary, Maryland, serious violent offenders including murderers and rapists can choose to participate in group and individual psychotherapy aimed at character reformation. The inmates are all recipients of indefinite (potentially lifelong) sentences, common among serious violent offenders in the United States, and seek therapy to secure an early release. When the therapy is successful, the parole board may grant the prisoner/patients early release if they are judged "better" and hence safe to leave. Assuming that it is not unjust to send murderers and rapists to prison for long, sometimes indefinite, periods, there seems to be no serious moral objection, deriving from the prisoners' rights, to the Patuxent prisoners being offered therapy. It is true that the choice as to whether to enter the programme is constrained by the fact that the alternative is to spend a very long time, possibly life, in prison; but, unlike the choice of "your money or your life" which a highwayman offers his victim, this is not unjust, unless the prisoner/patients were *unjustly* sentenced to long-term imprisonment in the first place. First, their necessarily limited choices are extended by being offered psychotherapy. Second, they can always leave the programme and return to the conventional state penitentiary to serve their term. Finally, the therapy offered is designed to give them greater emotional autonomy—to enable them to understand and rationally control their violent antisocial tendencies—a project in which they are willing participants. The more compelling objections to the Patuxent programme do not arise from fears about an all-encompassing psychotherapeutic state. Rather they arise from doubts about the efficacy of the therapy and fears that patient/prisoners, through pretending to have reformed, will be released prematurely, thus endangering the public. Indeed, one prisoner was released early and within a short time had committed another violent crime. This is a legitimate worry, but one that lies outside our present discussion. The principle that justifies psychotherapy as an alternative to long prison sentences is one of minimal restriction of liberty. Therapists participating in such a programme may legitimately argue that the scheme benefits patient and society alike: there is no conflict of interest, so no attendant moral dilemma.

In discussing problems concerning the use of therapy in coercive contexts, it is vital to distinguish between the question of whether it is right to offer therapy at all in such contexts, and that of whether particular types of therapy are justifiable. Of concern to defenders of civil liberties is the use of behaviour therapy in prisons. In the early 1970s, the Patuxent programme was, in fact, condemned for using "segregation cells", apparently as part of behaviour therapy for those on the therapeutic programme. A judicial hearing in 1971 held that the physical conditions in the segregation cells constituted "cruel and unusual punishment" and were, as such, illegal. Of all the psychotherapies, behaviour therapy most closely resembles non-psychological therapies such as drug therapy, and on this account it especially alarms Szasz and other libertarians. Unlike analytic therapy, behaviour therapy *can* be imposed on unwilling patients. Such therapy works by manipulating the patient's environment in such a way as to cause the patient to substitute desirable for undesirable behaviour. In itself, behaviour therapy is no more morally problematic than any other therapy. Although what constitutes "desirable" behaviour may be socially defined, behaviour therapy usually *does* aim to give the patient more control over her own behaviour and thus more autonomy, and, if it works, this is fine for the patient.

In evaluating behaviour therapy in prisons and other coercive contexts, it is necessary to make distinctions between the different ways in which it can be used. The least problematic is where the prisoner *consents* to a *positive* reinforcement schedule. The basis of this is the rewarding of desirable behaviour. The prisoner will never be made worse off than she would have been had she not joined the programme, and such treatments do not raise further moral difficulties since they are carried out with the prisoner's consent and cause the prisoner no extra pain, suffering, or other harm.

More problematic are cases where prisoners are subjected, whether they agree or not, to programmes involving a "token economy" and "time out" for misconduct, an extreme version of which is the segregation cells condemned at Patuxent. Under these programmes, prisoners' access to money or tobacco may be restricted if their behaviour is unsatisfactory, or they may be compelled to spend time in solitary confinement, all of which is likely to cause them at least some pain and suffering, and be experienced as degrading. Such treatments raise two problems. First, they may be carried out without the prisoner's consent, sometimes against her will. Second, they may require the inmate to suffer more deprivation than is warranted by the custodial sentence itself. In 1980, a joint working party of the Royal College of Psychiatrists, the Royal College of Nursing, and the British Psychological Society published a report, whose brief was to formulate ethical guidelines for behaviour modification therapy in the British National Health Service (HMSO, 1980). The report expressed concern about the use of negative reinforcement schedules, arguing that as a general rule they should not be used even on voluntary patients, except with their express written consent.

The situation with prisoners is, however, not so straightforward. This was recognized by the authors of the report (although, having acknowledged the problem, they do not offer guidelines for a solution):

> People in default of the law, whether in any form of legal detention or offered probation with conditions of residence and treatment, need special consideration. It is known that the use of behaviour modification methods generally throughout an institution has been proposed and this, if given effect, would raise special questions relevant to consent, more especially if alternative forms of treatment were not readily available. The validity of consent would be further prejudiced where the only choice available to the contracting individual lay between prison and treatment by behaviour modification as a condition of probation.
> [HMSO, 1980]

There is a problem about ensuring that a prisoner's consent to treatment is genuine when the only alternative is a longer, or even indefinite, prison sentence. But prisoners, unlike voluntary patients, are by definition not at liberty. There is a need for clear guidelines as to what sorts of programmes are acceptable and what sorts of restrictions may be placed upon prisoners, and for a clear system of accountability. Mild aversion therapy, as part of an overall behaviour modification programme, most of which uses positive reinforcement, may well be consistent with proper respect for the individual, but there are readily imaginable programmes that are not.

To take an extreme fictional case: in Anthony Burgess's novel *A Clockwork Orange*, the hero Alex, a pathologically violent young man, is sentenced to fourteen years in jail after committing numerous attacks on innocent people, and ultimately murder. Two years into his sentence, having been beaten up by warders and subjected to brutal prison conditions, he is given the opportunity of release within a matter of weeks if he agrees to be subjected to "Ludovico's Treatment". Not surprisingly, Alex is happy to volunteer. Ludovico's treatment is a fairly crude form of aversion therapy. Alex is strapped into a chair, with his eyes held open so that he cannot avoid watching a screen on to which are projected scenes of great violence. At the same time, music from Beethoven's Ninth Symphony is played to Alex (Beethoven's music, his favourite, for some reason stirs him to be violent). Just before the film and music start, Alex is injected with a strong emetic, so that as the music starts to excite him to have thoughts of violence he is acutely sick. This procedure is repeated several times. The result of this behaviour therapy is that whenever Alex has thoughts of violence he suffers from acute nausea. His violent behaviour is firmly "under control", although not in an autonomy-enhancing way, and he is safely returned to society. But in the novel, Alex's release is disastrous for him. The society in which he lives is exceptionally violent, and he is now unable to defend himself from attack by other people. Whenever he thinks of fighting back, he is overcome with nausea. Ultimately, the treatment is reversed as a result of public outrage and political pressure.

The reader might think that this example from fiction is irrelevant because such a treatment would never be inflicted on an inmate. For one thing, any treatment as crude as Ludovico's is unlikely to work in the long run. However, it is not so very far from this real case cited by Szasz:

Three convicted child molesters have sued to end a state program which uses electric shock and social conditioning to change their sex behaviour. The three inmates say the program is unconstitutional because they are allegedly forced to participate to gain parole. As part of the program's therapy shock is administered to the groin during a slide show of nude children. The shock stops when slides of nude women are shown. [Szasz, 1979]

Happily, such treatments are not commonly used, not least because they are now widely thought to be inefficacious. The objection put forward by counsel for the inmates was not to the therapy itself, but to the fact that accepting it was made a condition of parole. There are, however, two possible problems here. First, it may be thought that the treatment itself is inhuman and degrading. If it were so, then consent to it by the prisoners would not justify inflicting it upon them. Second, there is a suggestion not just that the prisoners could expect early parole if they agreed to the treatment, but that a refusal to agree to it would mean that parole would be delayed beyond the time when they could have expected to be released were it not for the treatment. The inmates are not literally forced to undergo the treatment, in that it takes place only with their written consent. However, doubt must be cast on the validity of such consent, which seems to be demanded under conditions of duress. We believe that any treatment programme that inflicts severe pain or deprivation on a prisoner should be tried only with the prisoner's informed consent, only as a last resort, when other, less invasive treatments have been tried, and never "offered" as a threat to make the prisoner worse off if she refuses the treatment than she would have been were the treatment unavailable.

Unless there are clear enforceable guidelines, and possibly legislation, restricting the conditions under which behaviour modification techniques may be used in prisons, and with compulsory psychiatric patients, there *is* a danger that therapy will be used, not for the benefit of the patient, but as an instrument of social coercion and control. One particular danger is that prisoners may effectively be threatened with *extra* punishment (over and above that "earned" through their criminal behaviour) unless they agree to undergo a therapeutic programme. Determination of the exact restrictions that should be placed on therapeutic programmes in prisons should not be left to individual therapists, who, as employees of the state and therapist for the patient, may be in a very compromising position. We believe that the use of threats to produce "consent" to therapy should be out-lawed, and that in any case therapists, of all people, should not participate in it. The imposition of negative reinforcement schedules on unwilling, socially deviant patient/prisoners evokes a revulsion weaker than, though reminiscent of, that produced by the Nazi doctors who carried out "experiments" on their unfortunate victims in concentration camps. Both therapists and patient/prisoners need protection.

Psychotherapy as an alternative to compulsory care orders for minors

It is not only within prisons that psychotherapists have an ethically ambiguous role as servants of both patient and the state authorities who employ them. Worries about psychotherapists being used as coercive agents of the state have also been expressed over the use of therapy, especially family therapy, with juveniles who have fallen foul of school, social services, or police authorities. In thinking about the use of therapy in such contexts, it is most important to appreciate that it raises genuine ethical dilemmas and not to be blinded by the rhetoric of those who think that it is either obviously wrong or obviously unproblematic.

THE GIRL WHO DID NOT LIKE SCHOOL

A 14-year-old girl had attended school on only twelve days in the previous two terms, in spite of her mother's efforts to persuade her to go. Her father had very little influence over his daughter and thought that sending her to school was the mother's responsibility. By an order of the court, the child was placed under the care of the local authority. Instead of being put in a children's home, she was admitted, with her own and her parents' consent, into the adolescent unit of a local hospital. After three weeks' intensive therapy, consisting mainly of family therapy with her parents and younger brother, she returned home and from then on attended school fairly regularly; the father took a greater interest in his daughter's education, and the girl even did well in her examinations.

Whereas some would not recognize that this use of therapy is even *prima facie* questionable, libertarians would strongly object to it. What, if anything, is wrong with it?

It *could* be objected that it is wrong for the girl to be regarded as in some way "ill" just because she refuses to submit to parental or school authority. To regard her rebelliousness as an illness dehumanizes her and stifles the possibility of freely expressing opposition to school and parental control.

However, as we have argued, to be a suitable case for psychotherapy does not entail that one be regarded as ill. There are many examples of people seeking, getting, and benefiting from psychotherapy, who are disturbed but are certainly neither ill nor regarded as such. In the case of the girl in our example, she failed to attend school because, in addition to finding lessons rather boring, she had a father who was apparently unconcerned and a mother who did not command her respect. None of the family wanted the girl to go into care, they all wanted family relationships to improve, and they all wanted, in so far as an opinion was expressed at all, the girl to do well in her examinations. By these criteria, the therapy certainly helped to achieve the family's goals, without any implication that the girl was ill, or simply an object for treatment.

A second objection is that the girl and her family were effectively being coerced into attending the family sessions, for the alternative—the girl remaining in care—was in their eyes so ghastly that they would do almost anything to prevent it. The consent is therefore no more valid than that of a highwayman's victim who hands over her money.

The situation is similar in certain respects to that of the prisoner who is faced with the choice between an invasive therapy and the completion of a long prison sentence. It is further complicated by the fact that the girl is a minor. In all the Western industrialized states, there is legislation designed to ensure that children receive proper education in school, unless the parents can provide a suitable alternative. One consequence of this is that the state has the authority to take a persistent truant into care to see that she does receive schooling. No doubt part of the rationale for this is to benefit the child, and part of it is to protect the public interest. The primary compulsion or coercion is in the legislation that insists that children should go to school. Offering family therapy to a girl who is already the subject of a care order, as a way of making it possible for her to avoid long-term removal from the family home, may actually increase her and her family's freedom. Instead of the child being forced to stay in care, it provides her with another option and therefore, through widened choice, *greater* autonomy. Admittedly, she has less liberty than she would have had if she could simply refuse to go to school and be left alone. But she has more liberty than had she not been offered therapy.

There are two aspects to the girl's freedom: the freedom or otherwise of her choice to enter therapy, and the increased freedom she could enjoy as a result of it. If the original choice is actually made freely and if the therapy actually would enhance her freedom, it is difficult to see how concern for the girl could lead to sound objections to family therapy in such a case. In many of these circumstances, the therapist may serve both the education authority and the child: their interests do not conflict. But there remains the need to place restrictions on what sorts of therapies and methods of persuasion should be permissible. As in the case of psychotherapy in prisons, this should not be left entirely to the discretion of individual therapists. There is a need for clear enforceable guidelines, particularly to ensure that programmes are explained to families as fully as is practicable, and that they are only embarked upon when they are genuinely the least coercive option available for a child.

A third objection is that putting therapists in the role of agents of the state (in our example, ensuring that the girl attends school) is arguably an abuse of their role as healers of the distressed. Szasz, for example, writes the following:

> In language and law, cure and control are like two banks of a river clearly separated by a body of water—that is, they are clearly separated by a willingness to distinguish between the interests of two parties in conflict with each other. The word *therapy*—as in psychiatric therapy or behaviour therapy—is a bridge over the water: it unites the two parties in a fake cooperation and enables one or the other or both of them to declare the non-existence of any difference between cure and control, contract and coercion, freedom and slavery. [Szasz, 1979]

Implicit in this is the view that therapists ought to be helping cure people, not, as in this case, controlling them. We have already touched on this in our discussion of behaviour therapy in prisons. It is wrong for people who are supposed to be healers to work as producers of social conformity.

Let us assume that the objector is not complaining about the Education Acts that make attendance at school compulsory, for this is not at issue here. If it is acceptable for the state to compel reluctant children to attend school, there are two plausible objections to therapists persuading children and their parents to have therapy instead of the child being taken into care, and to giving them therapy under these conditions. The first is that to do so would be deceitful—pretending that they are the patient's advocate and protector, when really they are primarily the agent of the state. The second is that asking therapists so clearly to act as agents of social policy, rather than as advocates of their patients, puts them in an impossible, hopelessly compromised, position and may weaken the integrity of all psychotherapists as defenders and promoters of personal autonomy.

The problem of deception is, in principle, superable. A family therapist could explain to the child and her family that they are being invited to family sessions primarily because the law insists that the child attends school. After all, a precondition of autonomy is facing up to reality, and psychotherapy can help patients face reality without necessarily endorsing it. As with the use of psychotherapy in prisons, it is important that the child's therapist explain at the outset—as fully as the circumstances, including the child's developmental stage, allow—what the aims and methods of the therapy are, as well as its likely effects, and what alternatives are available. There is a need to protect children from being brow-beaten by over-zealous therapists.

The fear about the integrity of psychotherapists may be easier to allay than might at first appear. As we have stressed repeatedly, there are many different types of therapy and therapist. There is no reason to suppose that the more behaviourally based treatment programmes that are used by adolescent units or prison units will undermine therapies or therapists operating in different contexts. The problems of therapists possibly being compromised are similar to those encountered by other enforcers of the law. They are encountered equally by social workers, probation officers, teachers, prison doctors, and so on. The main need is to recognize that this is an occupational hazard, and to provide support and protection for people working in these areas. Although it can be distressing for individuals to work in these coercive conditions, they should be given credit for providing a service to people who would otherwise be abandoned to more custody and less freedom.

In principle the use of psychotherapy in coercive institutions or settings is not worse than the primary coercion, or threat of it, that vitiates a patient's consent. Psychotherapy in such contexts should be banned only if it is impossible to provide strong safeguards against its abuse. There is a need for firm restrictive guidelines to be laid down both for the kind of treatment offered and for the circumstances in which individuals come to have the treatment. Given the inevitable pressure that such a possible conflict of loyalties may generate, and particularly in view of the pressure that state agencies may put on a therapist to "get results", there is a need for institutional support to ensure that ethical standards are maintained, and that therapists are protected from undue pressure. The development of a unified psychotherapy profession, which we discuss in chapter ten, seems to us crucial to this objective.

Third-party rights: confidentiality

Many professional relationships are founded on the assumption that what passes between professional and client is a matter for them alone, and breaches of professional confidentiality are regarded as seriously unethical. This is true not just of medicine, but also of banking, accountancy, and the law. In these professions, it may be not only unethical for a professional to give away a secret that she has heard from a client, but also either illegal or against the code of practice of the profession.

There are many reasons for regarding confidentiality in a professional relationship as vital. The most telling have to do with the fact that the professional, in order to help a client, must be given information that, for various reasons, the client would not want other people to discover.

If the professional could not guarantee confidentiality, many clients who need help simply would not seek it, or would give their professional helpers incomplete information. If this happened on a wide scale, it would lead to disastrously worse decisions being made by ill-informed professionals.

Furthermore, it is widely accepted that people have a right to privacy in their own personal affairs. This right stems from the fact that having control over the disclosure of personal information is partially constitutive of the basic freedom of choice over one's own relationships with other people. Ensuring professional confidentiality is a way of protecting this right.

Finally, the whole institution of professional help for clients is predicated on the assumption that the professional helper will act as the agent of the client. I employ my lawyer to act on my behalf, not just to see that, *from a neutral point of view*, the best decision is reached in a case. The professional, in accepting the role of my agent, is supposed to act as I would, if I had her expert knowledge or special skill. I may instruct someone to handle the negotiations concerning the purchase of a house for me. I employ her because of her legal expertise. Just as I, were I acting for myself, would not disclose to the sellers the limits of my financial resources, so I would expect my lawyer not to do so either, without my permission.

It is widely accepted that to reveal *without permission to a third party any* information one has received in confidence is a breach of trust and hence *prima facie* wrong. For professionals to breach professional confidences is, according to most codes of ethics, unacceptable. All individuals, and professionals in particular, do, however, have responsibilities not only to those who may give them confidential information, but also to others in their society. There may be a direct conflict between maintaining a confidence and protecting the legitimate interests of others. Such dilemmas could crop up within any profession. A banker, for example, may discover from confidential information that the money in a customer's deposit account is the proceeds of a heroin racket. Should she report the depositor to the police? Her duty of confidence conflicts with her duty to protect the public from heroin gangsters. Probably the moral duty to protect the public from the scourge of the heroin trade should prevail, although this would not, perhaps, be obvious to a banker in Switzerland, where the success of the banking business depends on confidence that bankers will *never* betray secret information about their clients or their accounts. A doctor may know, through confidential records, that a patient of hers suffers from epileptic fits. If she learns that the patient has just become a long-distance lorry driver, obviously not having declared her epilepsy, there is again a clear conflict of duties concerning whether or not she should inform the police or the licensing authorities. Given the possible horrendous consequences of a lorry driver blacking out while driving, most would argue that in these circumstances the information should be revealed to protect the public.

Different professional organizations have different ethical guidelines for their members, although all regard confidentiality as very important. In searching for limits to the duty of professional confidentiality, it is necessary to look beyond the particular situation of an individual professional faced with a dilemma to the kind of profession in which he or she works, and the role that confidentiality plays within it.

The professionals who are given most protection by the courts against revealing professionally acquired information are lawyers. Although the secrets revealed to lawyers by their clients do not necessarily contain the most intimate details of the clients' lives, the role of lawyers as advocates puts them in a special position. The adversarial system of justice requires that both parties should be able to present the strongest case possible. The peculiar role of lawyers as advocates would be severely undermined if they were forced or even permitted to reveal what they were told in private by clients. Many lawyers believe that under no circumstances should they disclose confidential information given to them by clients. Although this could in a particular case lead to great hardship—for example, the long imprisonment or even execution of an innocent person—these lawyers believe that, unless the protection of confidences is absolute, dangerous inroads will be made into the whole judicial process, weakening institutions that overall serve the interests of clients and the public alike.

On the other hand, although as a rule doctors must respect confidentiality, they may be required to reveal confidential information, and it is widely recognized within the medical profession that a doctor's responsibility to society may, *in extremis,* make breaking a confidence the right thing to do. The British Medical Association's *Handbook of Medical Ethics* states as follows:

> A doctor, like any other citizen, is a member of society with all the responsibilities this entails. Occasions may arise in which these persuade the doctor that information acquired in the course of medical consultation must be disclosed. In line with the principles of medical secrecy, whenever possible the doctor should seek to persuade the patient to disclose the information himself or give permission for the doctor to disclose it. Failing this, it will be for the doctor and for his own conscience to decide on his further course of action. [British Medical Association, 1981]

What about confidentiality within psychotherapy? Confidentiality within psychotherapy is special, because of the peculiar nature of the therapeutic relationship, which we described in chapter six. It has features in common with that between doctor and patient, parent and child, confessor and confessant (where the duty of confidentiality is often regarded as absolute), and advocate and client—and yet it is not entirely like any of these.

The subject-matter of psychotherapy includes fantasies, fears, and feelings that patients find very hard to acknowledge, even to themselves, let alone to anyone to whom their therapists might choose to talk. Most patients find Freud's "basic rule" hard enough in itself, and without a particularly strong expectation of confidentiality it is likely that many would become even more inhibited in the exploration of their psyches. This, in turn, would make it harder still for them to reach, with their therapists, the root of their problems. Psychotherapy is unique in that its subject-matter includes those areas of a patient's life which are most secret, often kept, by defence mechanisms, even from the patient's own awareness.

As mentioned in chapter one, psychotherapy is a medium where the normal rules of social encounters are suspended, and where it is safe to regress at times into kinds of behaviour that would be quite inappropriate in another setting. This feeling of safety requires a strong understanding that what goes on in therapy is strictly between therapist and patient.

Because of social prejudice against people suffering from psychological distress, there can be a stigma attached to going to a therapist. This provides a good reason why not only the contents of a therapeutic relationship but also the *fact* of such a relationship should be regarded as a matter of confidentiality.

There are then, rather as in the case of lawyers, good reasons for believing that the principle of respecting confidentiality in therapy should be very strong indeed. Without such an assumption, most psychotherapy would be impossible. It does not follow from this, however, that there should be an *absolute* ban on therapists revealing to others what they have been told in confidence by their patients. Indeed, as we shall see, the courts have held that the duty of confidence to patients is strictly limited, as in the case of doctors, by a duty to society as a whole. Are the courts right, and, if so, where should the limits of confidentiality for therapists be drawn? The issue is complicated and needs more detailed discussion. Many of these issues are raised clearly by a well-known tragic case, where a therapist's failure to warn a young woman that his patient had expressed a desire to kill her contributed to her being murdered.

THE TARASOFF CASE

On 27 October 1969, Prosenjit Poddar killed his former girl-friend Tatiana Tarasoff. Two months before doing so, Poddar had confided to his therapist that he wanted to kill Tarasoff when she returned to California after spending the summer in Brazil. Poddar was a voluntary out-patient at the Cowell Memorial Hospital at the University of California, Berkeley. At his therapist's request, the police detained Poddar for questioning. However, they subsequently released him as he appeared rational, denied any intention to kill Tarasoff, and undertook to stay away from her. When the matter was referred back to the Director of Psychiatry at the hospital, he asked that the case be dropped and that the correspondence with the police be destroyed. Poddar did not return for more therapy, apparently because his therapist had breached confidentiality by informing the police. Two months later he went to Tatiana Tarasoff's home and shot and stabbed her to death.

Tarasoff's parents sued the therapist and his psychiatrist supervisor for negligence in failing to warn Tatiana or them of the danger that she was in. The Supreme Court of California ruled that the therapists were at fault, putting forward the maxim that "Protective privilege ends where public peril begins".

The Tarasoff case (*Tarasoff v. Regents of the University of California* [1976] 131 Cal RPTR. 14) has attracted much publicity, in part because it is so unusual, and it would be unwise to try to base recommendations for the future of psychotherapy on consideration of extreme and atypical cases alone. Nevertheless, the case does bring into sharp focus some of the conflicts that remain perhaps unclear and below the surface in everyday psychotherapy. The case has profound implications for professional secrecy in therapy ("*Tarasoff* Decision", 1987).

The Supreme Court of California held that psychotherapists have a legal duty of care to members of the public who are threatened by possible acts of violence by their patients. Once this is accepted, the victim or relatives of a victim of a violent attack by a patient have the chance to mount an action for negligence against a therapist who fails to reveal to the intended victim a patient's threats of violence. This judgement, which incidentally has not been followed in all states, has been strongly criticized by psychiatrists, who have maintained that the therapeutic relationship is seriously undermined by it, and that it is likely to be counter-productive.

With hindsight, it seems likely that the murder of Tarasoff could have been prevented had the therapists behaved differently. If Poddar's therapist had not gone to the police, Poddar might have stayed within therapy, and this could have led him to abandon his murderous intentions. On the other hand, if the therapist had insisted that the Tarasoff family be warned of the possible danger that they faced, Tatiana could, perhaps, have protected herself against the fatal attack.

It was argued that the therapists should have realized the seriousness of Poddar's threats, and that in not informing Tarasoff's family they were negligent. But the main legal question was not whether or not they were *careless*, but whether or not they owed a *duty of care* to Tarasoff and her family, and indeed to any member of the public who might have been threatened by their patient.

Prior to the Tarasoff ruling, it was widely held that a therapist was not under a duty to reveal confidential statements in order to protect a third party, and that the decision whether or not, in these circumstances, to break confidence should be a matter of personal conscience. Although it is clear that therapists have a duty of care to their patients, it was held that they had no general duty of care to the public in respect of the conduct of their patients.

The Tarasoff judgement has been criticized by psychiatrists on several grounds (Lane & Spruill, 1980; Karasu, 1981). They have held that it places therapists in an impossible legal position. Therapists are in danger of facing legal proceedings for breach of confidence—for example, in a situation where a threat of violence was *not*, as it turned out, genuinely intended. On the other hand, the Tarasoff ruling means that they may face legal proceedings if they do *not* break confidences. Given the intrinsic unpredictability of human actions, this is an unfair burden to place on therapists.

It has also been argued that if therapists can be under a legal obligation to reveal confidential information, this may have unwelcome side-effects that would heavily outweigh the benefits of protecting the occasional victim of patient violence. If patients realize, so it is argued, that therapists are under an obligation to disclose confidential information in cases where they believe that this reveals a serious threat to the safety of a member of the public, they may be deterred from entering therapy at all or, if they do enter therapy, are likely to be undesirably inhibited in what they reveal to the therapist, thus reducing the effectiveness of the therapy. In particular, if a patient has felonious intentions (which perhaps could be changed by therapeutic examination), she is unlikely to discuss them with a therapist who could be under a legal obligation to reveal what she has been told. Consequently, there is a danger that in the long run more people will be the victims of violent assault. There are potentially violent patients who could be helped by therapy to overcome their feelings of violence, but only by exploring those feelings thoroughly and openly. The Tarasoff ruling may mean that such people will not seek therapy and will therefore be more likely to commit acts of violence. There is a danger that the decision will be counterproductive even in its own terms.

It is difficult to evaluate the factual assumptions of these consequentialist arguments. Sissela Bok remains sceptical:

> No evidence suggests that therapy will be imperilled if patients know that therapists have the duty to reveal their plans of violence. Even if therapy were thus imperilled, it is not clear that more violence would result. Not only have such contentions not been proved; many doubt that they are even probable. Patients rarely place much trust in confidentiality regarding their most extreme statements anyway, and may even hope that their threats *will* lead to some preventive action. [Bok, 1986]

Indeed, it can plausibly be argued that successful therapy requires that the therapist should not be bound by any *absolute* restriction of confidentiality imposed by the patient. Far from being counter-therapeutic, a therapist's maintaining the freedom to resist coercion and manipulation by the patient's neuroses may provide a model for the patient's own liberation.

THE PATIENT WITH THE COERCIVE MOTHER

A patient—an unhappy and dissatisfied woman in her 60s—told her therapist at the start of therapy that she had a secret that she would reveal only if he would guarantee absolute confidentiality. She hinted that it concerned medical negligence. The therapist assured her that the normal rules of confidentiality would be observed but, possibly rather perversely, questioned whether absolute confidentiality was possible. What if she blurted something out in her sleep, or inadvertently referred to the incident without thinking? The patient was infuriated by this response but did eventually reveal the episode, which, as is common in such situations, did not turn out to be particularly scandalous or dramatic. However, the therapist's instinctive refusal seemed to have beneficial results. The patient became less in thrall to her elderly mother, who insisted that she rang three times a day and made it impossible for her to go away even for a night. She also became more able to stand up to the demands of her adolescent daughter.

Accepting that therapists should have discretion as to whether to reveal confidences is a rather different matter from making it a legal *obligation* for them to disclose threats to the public which have been revealed in confidence by their patients. There is a fear that such an obligation would push therapists too far towards becoming agents of society rather than of their individual patients (Lakin, 1988). This could, for example, generate particularly severe role conflicts for psychotherapists working in prisons. Once the principle of requiring therapists to reveal confidences in some circumstances has been established, it may be difficult to impose satisfactory limits on these requirements. It is one thing for therapists to recognize a duty to protect the public, quite another for them to be put in a position where they have to become an adjunct to the police force.

A further argument for therapists having an absolute privilege not to have to reveal confidences gained by them from patients is that to break a therapeutic confidence is a direct assault on the patient's autonomy, which it is the therapist's job to enhance and protect. This sort of argument is, however, given short shrift by Bok:

> The autonomy we grant individuals over personal secrets, first of all, cannot reasonably be thought to extend to plans of violence against innocent persons; at such times, on the contrary, someone who knows of plans that endanger others owes it to them to counteract those plans, and, if he is not sure he can forestall them, to warn the potential victims. Nor, in the second place, can

patients who voice serious threats against innocent persons in-
voke confidentiality on the basis of their relationship with therapists or anyone else without asking them to be partially
complicitous. [Bok, 1986]

In cases where a therapist faces a genuine conflict of interests
between a patient and potential victims of the patient, it is impossible
to act fully in the interests of both. Accepting a patient for therapy
gives the therapist a special responsibility for the patient. But there is
no reason why this responsibility should eclipse a general responsibility to others not to collude in violence against them. Even parents
have a moral duty to protect innocent victims from assaults by their
children.

In our discussion of manipulation and deception within therapy,
we argued that they could be justified as being in the patient's interests when they are autonomy-enhancing. Here, the breaking of
confidences can be justified—even though it is a violation of respect
for the patient's autonomy—when it is necessary to protect in the
most vital way the autonomy of an intended victim of violence. In
such circumstances, *someone's* autonomy must be compromised, and,
given that the patient has already repudiated respect for her intended
victim's autonomy, it might be wrong for the therapist to sacrifice the
innocent victim to protect the patient, notwithstanding the special
relationship between therapist and patient.

If occasions may arise where it would be morally wrong for a
therapist *not* to divulge a confidence, therapists should be very wary,
as most therapists in fact are, of making categorical promises that
they will never, under any circumstances, disclose information given
them in confidence. Therapists should not lose sight of their moral
duties of common humanity to fellow citizens who are not their patients.

On the other hand, it is not clear that using legal sanctions to
attempt to force therapists to disclose certain confidences is the best
way of protecting the interests of those affected. Such sanctions may,
as has been suggested, prove counter-productive. Making failure to
disclose a *criminal* offence would seriously compromise the therapist's independence and, for the reasons given above, would be
unlikely to reduce assaults by psychotherapy patients. On the other
hand, to render therapists who fail to disclose confidential information to threatened parties liable for the civil wrong of negligence is

also fraught with problems. The recent expansion in medical litigation has had a disastrous effect on the quality and availability of care for patients in the United States: doctors' indemnity rates have soared, there has been a massive increase in defensive medicine, and in certain states doctors are reluctant to practise as neurosurgeons or obstetricians for fear of litigation. The result is that medical insurance for patients is more expensive, and there is a shortage of good doctors in vital areas; it is by no means clear that overall medical practice has improved as a result.

If therapists were obliged through fear of criminal or civil proceedings to disclose confidential information to threatened third parties, it is not obvious that the Prosenjit Poddars of this world would reveal their murderous intentions to their therapists. Legal sanctions would probably not prevent tragedies such as that which befell Tatiana Tarasoff, and the unintended side-effects of such sanctions would be very costly.

One of the major reasons for having sympathy with the Tarasoff judgement is the thought that Tarasoff's family *should* be compensated for their tragic loss, although no compensation could be adequate, and that unless the therapists were held to be liable for negligence they would have no remedy. A solution to this problem would be to implement a no-fault accident compensation scheme such as exists in New Zealand. Victims of "accidents", which include injuries caused by sheer bad luck, negligence, or deliberate violence, are compensated from a national fund paid for out of taxation. It is not necessary to prove that someone is to blame in order for victims to be compensated.

Once compensation is separated from the need to prove fault, much of the case for making disclosure of confidential information by therapists a *civil* legal obligation falls away. The majority of therapists would, in an emergency, be prepared to break a confidence to save a victim from violent assault. The difficult cases, such as that faced by Poddar's therapist, are matters of the finest judgement, largely to do with the therapist's assessment of the likelihood of the patient carrying out the threat; and the law is, of necessity, a blunt instrument.

The other main reason for having a fault-based system of tort liability is to deter practitioners from bad practice. We have, however, argued that in the area in question to impose a duty of care on therapists to disclose threats of violence made by patients, to their intended victims, is unlikely to produce the desired effect. Perhaps a better way of encouraging good practice among therapists would be for there to be clear professional guidelines both about when breaches of confidence are permissible or required, and about how, if at all, an anticipated breach should be communicated to the patient. Failure to follow a code of practice could result in professional disciplinary proceedings. As with defining precisely the goals of therapy at the outset, there would be a problem if therapists were required to declare at the start of therapy exactly what the conditions were under which confidence might be breached. If the therapist declares that she might break a confidence if she thinks the patient is likely to commit a felony or seriously harm herself, this very statement might inhibit therapy, as it could be interpreted as arising out of the specific relationship with *this* patient, rather than being a requirement of the code of practice. Perhaps the best compromise solution to this problem would be to make these guidelines, or a shortened version of them, readily available to all psychotherapy patients and to encourage patients to read them.

In reality, it is rare for psychotherapy patients actually to carry out threats of violence against others, rather less so in the case of threats against themselves. To have an expectation of confidentiality, except in cases where the therapist believes that maintaining confidence would constitute a serious danger, would be unlikely seriously to deter those who needed therapy from seeking it. The danger of deterring potential patients could be reduced further if therapists agreed not to divulge confidences without first discussing the proposed disclosure with the patient, giving the patient an opportunity to present a case against disclosure.

The general principle underlying the limits of confidentiality should be that confidential information given to a therapist by a patient in therapy is the property of the patient, and should not be divulged to a third party unless this is judged by the therapist to be necessary for the protection of someone's safety. It would, of course, be a matter of argument exactly what was meant by "necessary for the protection of someone's safety". Furthermore, a therapist who intends to break a confidence should, wherever practicable, seek the consent of the patient and at least discuss the proposed breach of confidentiality with the patient. The principle of no revelation without consultation should, however, not be *absolute*. It is implicit in all these principles that there *could* be extreme situations where the principle would have to be abandoned—for example, where the patient is armed, dangerous, threatening imminent violence, and in no mood to talk about anything.

If a protocol such as that proposed above were incorporated within a professional code of practice, it would be possible for disciplinary proceedings to be brought against offending therapists. We think that such proceedings, carried out by a professional body, are likely to be more effective in protecting the interests of all concerned than having such lapses litigated in the courts.

Conclusion

In this chapter, we have discussed three key areas where therapists may find themselves facing conflicting responsibilities—to their patients, and to society at large. There is no neat or straightforward solution to these problems. On the one hand, the special relationship between therapist and patient needs to be protected; on the other, therapists should not lose sight of the fact that they are members of a broader society, with the attendant responsibilities of such membership.

There are two kinds of problem here: what constitutes ethically acceptable practice, and how it is best promoted. We have made suggestions about what would constitute good practice. As to the problems of promoting good practice, and protecting the public from bad practice, we have expressed scepticism about the efficacy of tackling them through civil or criminal legislation. On the other hand, there are many reasons why the matter should not simply be left to the conscience of individual practitioners. In the next two chapters, we consider proposals for tackling the problem of practitioner compliance and for ensuring that patients and the public receive a psychotherapy service of the highest ethical and technical standards.

CHAPTER 9

Ethical codes
and codes of practice
in psychotherapy

If, as we argued in the previous chapter, both simple appeal to therapists' consciences *and* attempted direct control by legislation are unsatisfactory vehicles for minimizing incompetent or unconscionable conduct among therapists, the most obvious alternative is for some regulation from within the body of psychotherapists itself. The medical profession has attempted to regulate its own professional standards at least since the fourth century BC when the Hippocratic Oath was formulated. Since the Second World War, several codes of medical ethics have been published, most notably the 1947 International Code of Medical Ethics following the Geneva Declaration of the World Medical Association, amended by the 22nd World Medical Assembly held in Sydney, Australia, in 1968.

As psychotherapy has expanded, so ethical problems arising out of therapy have become one of the central issues for the nascent profession. Our discussions in the previous three chapters have shown how the therapist has special moral responsibilities, and inevitably faces tough moral dilemmas. There is therefore a need for considerable moral integrity among therapists.

If the monitoring and promotion of good standards is to come from within psychotherapy, the best way to achieve this, as we shall argue in detail in chapter ten, and as is being increasingly realized, would be for psychotherapy to become a recognized profession. One of the features of many professions, of which medicine is just one example, is the development of a professional code of ethics.

The main questions addressed in this chapter are: what are the special features of codes of ethics in psychotherapy, and would the development of a code of psychotherapeutic ethics be likely to make a significant contribution to solving moral dilemmas within psychotherapy, and to ensuring high moral standards among its practitioners?

Special responsibilities and codes of ethics

According to most moral theories, morality consists of a set of principles that apply to *everyone*, irrespective of their particular position or status. Lying, cheating, and violent assault, for example, are immoral whether one is an accountant, a doctor, or a civil servant. Moral principles are, it seems, universal.

In view of this, someone might ask: "What is the point of an ethical code for any particular group of people?" Surely, the argument goes, everyone is bound by ethical principles, so there can be no specific ethics for a particular group, whether or not its members form a professional association. There are no distinctively *medical* ethics. There is therefore no reason to have a distinctive *code* of medical ethics.

The obvious rejoinder to this sceptical assault on the very idea of a professional code of ethics is to point out that different groups of people may have different special responsibilities. Parents, for example, have special responsibilities for their own children, citizens for their own community, and professionals for their clients and the good standing of their profession. Arising out of these special responsibilities, one could envisage the development of "parenting ethics", "citizenry ethics", and various kinds of "professional ethics". These would not be defining new fundamental principles, as if parents could employ different moral principles from other people. Rather, they would concentrate, using *general* ethical principles, on the special problems that are likely to be relevant to parenting.

Medical ethics uses general ethical principles to discuss moral problems that arise within and as a result of medical practice. Medical practitioners have felt that the role of doctors is sufficiently unlike that of other professionals for there to be a need for a specific code of medical ethics which should guide all doctors. We have argued that the therapeutic relationship is unique, and that this creates special responsibilities and dilemmas for the therapist. Is there, then, a good case for a specific code of ethics for psychotherapy?

The International Code of Medical Ethics: a test case

In order to answer this question it is instructive to examine the International Code of Medical Ethics, which was approved by the World Medical Assembly in 1968. We use it here as a basis of comparison for a possible code of psychotherapeutic ethics. The Code is divided into three sections: Duties of Doctors in General; Duties of Doctors to the Sick; and Duties of Doctors to Each Other. The first section declares that doctors must always maintain the highest standards of professional conduct, must not be motivated by profit, must not advertise without express authorization, and must receive no money for services rendered, except where this is a "proper professional fee". It declares that treating a patient in a way that weakens her physical or mental resistance is unethical, except where to do so is in the patient's interests. It advises against the injudicious disclosure of new discoveries, and against issuing certificates in the absence of personal verification by the doctor.

The third section declares that doctors ought to treat each other as they would have other doctors treat them, that they must not entice patients from colleagues, and finally that they must observe the principles of the *Declaration of Geneva*, which was approved by the World Medical Association and incorporated within the Code (as amended by the 22nd World Medical Assembly, Sydney, Australia, August 1968: see British Medical Association, 1981). The *Declaration is* a modern version of the ancient Hippocratic Oath. It includes the following:

> At the time of being admitted as a Member of the Medical Profession:
>
> I solemnly pledge myself to consecrate my life to the service of humanity;
>
> I will practise my profession with conscience and dignity;

The health of my patient will be my first consideration;

I will respect the secrets which are confided in me, even after the patient has died;

I will maintain by all the means in my power, the honour and the noble traditions of the medical profession;

My colleagues will be my brothers [sic];

I will not permit considerations of religion, nationality, race, party politics or social standing to intervene between my duty and my patients;

I will maintain the utmost respect for human life from the time of conception; even under threat, I will not use my medical knowledge contrary to the laws of humanity. [British Medical Association, 1981]

The duties of doctors to the sick, outlined in the second section of the Code, are characterized as follows:

A doctor must always bear in mind the obligation of preserving human life.

A doctor owes to his patient complete loyalty and all the resources of his science. Whenever an examination or treatment is beyond his capacity he should summon another doctor who has the necessary ability.

A doctor shall preserve absolute secrecy on all he knows about his patients because of the confidence entrusted in him.

A doctor must give emergency care as a humanitarian duty unless he is assured that others are willing and able to give such care. [British Medical Association, 1981]

One thing that is striking about the International Code of Medical Ethics is its enormous range. It includes both very general injunctions to maintain the highest standards of professional conduct, and the very specific requirement for a doctor to call on another doctor with the necessary ability whenever an examination or treatment is beyond his own capacity. The Code does define some of the special responsibilities of doctors—notably, to be committed to the preservation of life and to the health of their patients. It singles out some special obligations that doctors have to their patients: apart from the obligation to preserve human life, a commitment to bring all the resources of their science to the aid of their patients, a commitment to preserve absolute secrecy about the contents of dealings with their patients, and a general commitment not to deprive potential patients of emergency aid.

Such a code does, in our view, have a useful, but limited role to play. There are foreseeable contexts in which very general principles of the Code could have a significant use. For example, doctors could be asked by a repressive government to carry out a medical examination in order to ascertain whether or not a prisoner is fit to be subjected to torture. The principle in the *Declaration* stating that "The health of my patient will be my first consideration" could presumably rule out doctors undertaking such work. It is undesirable that doctors should be pressurized to carry out medical examinations that are not in the interests of their patients. Doctors will, on the whole, be able to make a more substantial contribution to humanity if they are protected from having to carry out certain tasks. The general principles of a code of ethics may offer such protection to individual doctors, and to prevent them from being used to legitimize the oppressive practices of tyrannical regimes.

On the other hand, the principle that states that doctors must maintain the highest standards of professional conduct is unlikely to help solve any practical problems, even though it may sound impressive. One key difficulty is that it leaves undefined what "the highest standards of professional conduct" might be. This is important since the matter could be controversial. Second, making it a requirement that doctors maintain the *highest* standards may in fact weaken the force of the whole code. Any doctor knows that not all doctors always maintain the highest standards, and that falling somewhat short of this ideal is, and is bound to be, tolerated by the profession. At best, such a principle is a helpful morale-booster, suggesting that doctors ought to be more devoted to the good of their patients than perhaps non-professionals need be to the good of those with whom they do business. Similarly, the injunction not to be influenced by motives of profit is just the sort of thing that it is easy to pay lip-service to and then safely ignore.

The specific recommendations regarding absolute secrecy—not enticing patients from colleagues, providing emergency care, and seeking expert help when a case is beyond the doctor's own competence—all at least have the virtue of determinacy and, consequent upon that, enforceability. There is a reasonable expectation that they will be taken seriously and will not be regarded just as pious principles, which can be safely ignored. However, they are not without difficulties.

One problem is that the Code, of necessity, singles out only a selection of specific recommendations, when there must be countless others that could be made. For example, the requirement that a doctor should "summon another doctor who has the necessary ability" in cases that are beyond his own competence would be accepted by most people on the grounds that it affords a basic protection to the patient. But so too would be the similar principle: "Senior doctors should not assign juniors to cases which, in the opinion of the senior, are beyond the competence of the junior." This principle is not included in the Code. Moreover, the principle of not exceeding one's professional competence in dealings with clients is general, and should apply, on the most general ethical principles, to any professional dealings. In reality, there are hundreds of specific principles that could arguably define good medical practice. A code of ethics that attempted to list all of them would be too long to be digestible and would, in any case, almost certainly fail to be comprehensive.

The supposed duties of doctors to the sick are interesting, because they do bring out some of the special features of the doctor's role, as compared with other professions. Whereas solicitors, accountants, and doctors all have special responsibilities for their own clients, doctors also have distinctive professional duties towards society at large. There are, however, serious moral difficulties with three of the supposed duties of doctors to the sick.

Doctors are told that they must always bear in mind the obligation of preserving human life. This suffers from vagueness, and it is doubtful whether it would help to solve many of the practical moral dilemmas that a doctor is likely to face. Consider, for example, the problem of an elderly, sick patient who wants to die, but could be kept alive by antibiotics.

The claim that doctors owe their patients complete loyalty might, if taken literally, mean that a doctor should give no weight to anyone else's needs. This is implausible and in any case could be inconsistent with both an obligation to preserve life and an obligation to provide emergency care, where this requires the temporary abandonment of a patient with a minor complaint.

There are serious problems, too, with the requirement that doctors "preserve absolute secrecy" on all information that they have learnt in confidence from their patients. In the previous chapter, we discussed problems associated with "absolute secrecy". There are cases where it would be wrong for a doctor not to reveal information given in confidence. We mentioned the case of the epileptic who becomes a long-distance lorry driver. Another example might be a doctor whose patient with AIDS is contemplating marriage without informing his fiancee.

The general moral of this is that doctors, like other people, have to confront a wide variety of different kinds of cases, and that simple principles such as "Do not reveal secrets", although good as general principles, are, as they stand, too simple and admit of too many exceptions. Acceptable exceptionless rules of conduct are likely to be either so detailed, because of disclaimers, as to be practically un-usable, or, like "always act according to the highest professional standards", so vague as to be of little practical relevance.

Before applying these considerations to the question of a possible code of ethics for psychotherapy, it is worth asking what a professional code of ethics should be for.

What is a professional code of ethics for?

One function of a code of ethics is to define, in the broadest terms, the special aims of a particular profession—the *raison d'être* of the profession. Doctors, for example, define their aims as the preservation of life and the promotion of the health of their patients. Barristers, on the other hand, have no special duties beyond those of ordinary citizens to preserve life or death, but they do have a duty to see that their clients are well-represented and perhaps to promote justice. Such statements have several functions: creating an atmosphere within the profession; promoting a public image of the profession; and offering individual members of the profession some protection from outside pressure to perform tasks that are inimical to their defined special responsibilities.

A second role of a code of ethics is to define certain standards of *ideal* conduct and attitude. In the case of the International Code of Medical Ethics, these would include such statements as that the doctor "will maintain by *all* [authors' italics] means in my power, the honour and the noble traditions of the medical professions", that doctors will always maintain the highest standards of professional conduct, and so on. As already pointed out, it cannot reasonably be expected that all doctors will adhere to such standards strictly, since this would require total dedication. These statements of ideal conduct have a very limited function. They are unenforceable, very vague, and, in so far as they *can* be given a determinate sense, do not pick out anything special about the profession in question. It is obvious that whereas it is desirable for any professional to maintain the highest professional standards, such ideal conduct will not always be adhered to by people who are nonetheless suitable to continue practising without penalty.

The third, and arguably most important, role of a code of ethics is to protect clients or patients from bad practice. This is achieved in part by making implicit ethical principles of professional responsibility explicit (British Association for Social Work, 1975). It requires that certain sorts of conduct are explicitly ruled out as unacceptable. This is the part of the code which has teeth and can be supported by sanctions. In the case of the International Code of Medical Ethics, receiving money other than a professional fee for services rendered is deemed unethical. Betraying confidences, treating patients beyond the doctor's competence, and failing to give emergency aid are also proscribed. These prohibitions have a number of functions. First, they offer some protection to members of the public against bad professional practice, because doctors who violate such prohibitions can be disciplined by the profession and even lose their registration and hence their licence to practise. Second, in common with statements of the special aims of a profession, they help to prevent outside bodies, such as governments, putting pressure on individual doctors to act in an unethical manner. Finally, by offering firm guidance they may help to relieve individual doctors of some of the burdens of moral dilemmas.

In assessing the worth of a code of ethics, it is important to distinguish these different parts and to look specifically at the function of each part. Declarations of ideal standards are not, and are probably not intended to be, enforceable against members, since their value lies, as we have suggested, in boosting morale and creating a certain atmosphere in the profession. However, a principle that was supposed to serve as a protection for the public against unconscionable professional practice would be seriously defective if it could not be enforced. One of the most serious limitations of ethical codes such as the International Code of Medical Ethics is that the various parts are jumbled up, and the language of requirement and compulsion is used in contexts where what is really being discussed is ideal conduct.

Should there be a code of ethics for psychotherapy?

As we have stressed, psychotherapists come from many different professions, including medicine, social work, and psychology, each of which has its own code of ethics. Perhaps the main argument against the idea of a separate code of ethics for psychotherapy is similar to an argument, to which we return in chapter ten, brought forward by clinical psychologists against a separate psychotherapy profession: that the professionals who practise psychotherapy are already members of professional bodies or associations, each of which has its own high standards and code(s) of ethics; there is therefore no need for either a distinct psychotherapy profession, or a distinct code of ethics.

This objection can be countered in two ways. First, not everyone who practises psychotherapy is a member of another recognized professional organization. Second, psychotherapy does have its own distinctive aims, and the psychotherapeutic relationship, although like other professional and personal relationships in certain respects, does have its own special features. A psychiatrist who is a doctor, and a psychologist who is not, may both practise psychotherapy. In so far as they are each practising psychotherapy the psychiatrist and psychologist will confront more problems common to each other's practice than would the doctor with non-psychotherapist doctors, or the psychologist with non-psychotherapist psychologists.

Assuming that the very idea of a code of ethics for psychotherapy is not outlandish, it is necessary to examine the issue in more detail by looking separately at the three different parts of a professional code of ethics which we identified above.

- *Statement of special aims:* We have argued throughout this book that one of the distinctive reasons for thinking psychotherapy valuable is its aim of enhancing patients' emotional autonomy. We have serious doubts about the efficacy of very general statements of ideals, such as the International Codes of Medical Ethics' "I solemnly pledge myself to consecrate my life to the service of humanity"; there is, however, some value in stating profession-specific aims. Just as medicine aims at health, and the legal profession at justice, so, in our view, psychotherapy aims at emotional autonomy. Such a declaration would probably have some limited value in creating a common identity for members of the psychotherapy profession, and would provide a very general standard by reference to which specific problem cases could be considered.

- *Statements of ideal standards:*   We have already expressed our scepticism about the value of such statements, apart from their limited effect on morale and professional atmosphere.

- *Specific prohibitions:*   This is the most important part of a code of ethics, since it is an attempt to protect clients of a professional service and could be accompanied by sanctions. We have argued that the psychotherapeutic relationship generates a special kind of dependency of the patient on the therapist. This gives the therapist a special moral responsibility, which this part of a code of ethics could help to uphold. For example, the temporary dependency that psychotherapy often creates can, as we have seen, be used by an unscrupulous therapist as a vehicle for exploiting a patient financially, sexually, or emotionally. There is also, arguably, a need to ensure that therapists are not used in contexts of coercion as agents of social control. Although we may assume that all professional abuse of clients is wrong, there could be a case for highlighting and specifically banning the sorts of abuse we have mentioned (financial or sexual exploitation of patients' psychological dependency, breaking confidences, imposition of degrading treatment on patients as a vehicle for social control, and so on), in order to protect both patients and therapists. The other principle for selecting specific prohibitions is that there are certain practices that, although perhaps discreditable in any relationship, are *normally* tolerable without sanction, but should *not* be, within the specific *professional* context.

No doubt these forms of patient abuse are by no means unique to psychotherapy, and there are certainly other moral crimes that could take place within a therapeutic relationship (murder would be an extreme example). But each of them picks out a form of abuse to which psychotherapy patients may be particularly vulnerable, and each identifies misdemeanours that, outside the context of psychotherapy, would be much less serious than within it.

A professional code of ethics for psychotherapy should include some statement of general principles to do with respect for the autonomy of everyone suffering from mental disturbance. It could also set out some features of good therapeutic practice: for example, that psychotherapists should always consider whether alternative forms of treatment to the one they are offering would be more beneficial to their patients, and, if they think so, should recommend the alternative.

But the most important role would be to define the boundaries of *acceptable* practice within the profession. In order to bring out some of the limitations of a code of ethics for psychotherapy, let us consider the following injunctions, which could plausibly find their way into such a code:

- A psychotherapist must not sexually exploit her/his patients.
- A psychotherapist must not financially exploit her/his patients.
- A psychotherapist must not deceive her/his patients.
- A psychotherapist must not reveal confidential information revealed to her/him by a patient.
- A psychotherapist must not engage in any "therapy" that is really just a covert form of policing.

Each of these prohibitions seems unexceptionable but contains serious difficulties either of interpretation or of plausibility, or of both.

Everyone can agree that sexual exploitation of patients by therapists is wrong. This is trivially true, since "exploitation", when used to describe a human relationship, is a term of condemnation. The serious problem that the statement leaves unanswered is: "How is sexual exploitation to be defined?" The limiting case would appear to be rape. But surely there should be no need to include a ban on rape as part of an ethical code for *psychotherapy*, any more than there should be a specific ban on murder, for this would suggest that outside a therapeutic relationship rape was not a serious crime. Is, then, any sexual contact between therapist and patient to count as sexual exploitation of the patient by the therapist? What if the contact takes place with the full consent of the patient, and does no harm? In chapter seven we argued that there was a good case for banning all sexual contact between therapist and patient. This was not, however, because all such contacts are necessarily exploitative or immoral but, rather, that partly for technical reasons a complete ban is likely best to promote the overall aims of therapy.

Rather than having a statement banning "sexual exploitation" of patients—a proscription with moral overtones—of more use would be a simple statement banning sexual contact, while a patient is in therapy, between therapist and patient. This, however, would leave untouched the vexed problem of therapist–patient sexual relationships after therapy has come to an end. As our discussion in chapter seven illustrates, this problem cannot be solved by a one-line moral injunction.

Financial exploitation raises similar problems. The main reason for thinking of including it in a code of psychotherapeutic ethics is that the very nature of psychotherapy creates a special danger of a patient being charged an exorbitant fee by a therapist, or being kept in therapy in inappropriate circumstances or for longer than is needed. The therapist may be paid a regular fee while the therapy is going nowhere and the patient remains dependent. But how is financial exploitation to be identified? There are two sides to it: charging too much, and treating inappropriately or for too long. The first problem could be solved by the profession agreeing to a scale of professional fees, but the second, as we have seen, is more intractable. For example, should a psychoanalyst be prevented from keeping in treatment a rich patient who wants to stay in analysis and is prepared to go on paying for it, even though the analyst realizes that the treatment is no longer helping the patient to achieve emotional autonomy and has, in fact, created a long-term dependency on the therapist? The psychoanalyst T. Reik describes how a millionaire offered, in return for a daily fifty-minute session, to pay him an enormous amount, which would have kept Reik in a luxurious lifestyle, enabling him to do all the writing he wanted (Reik, 1948). It was an attractive offer, but Reik reluctantly felt unable to accept, for fear that he would have been corrupted and would therefore have ended up exploiting his patient. But would it have been wrong for him to have taken this risk? Should he have been prevented from treating this patient on these terms, if both had wanted it? Again, for the prohibition of exploitation to be useful, there would need to be a detailed interpretation.

What about the principle banning deception within therapy? Everyone agrees that deception is wrong, although it may, in extreme circumstances, be justifiable—for example, when a crazed murderer asks you which way his intended victim has just gone. Something about deception would need to be included in a code of psychotherapeutic ethics because of the fiduciary nature of the therapeutic relationship. This is most clear in analytic psychotherapy, where the professed aim of the therapy is to enable patients to become more autonomous by coming to understand and accept the truth about what they are really like, painful and difficult though this may be. This requires patients to place enormous trust in their therapists and therefore makes them particularly vulnerable to manipulation and deception. Furthermore, there is a special temptation for therapists, in order to save time, to employ strategies that rely on deception.

However, the situation is far more complicated than the simple principle mentioned above might suggest. There is the by now familiar problem of interpretation: "What exactly is meant by deception?" This is particularly relevant within therapies that make use of paradox, where the therapist utters literal falsehoods as the most effective way of communicating deep-seated truths. In addition, there are likely to be rare occasions where deception is warranted. The limiting case of the crazed murderer could occur within therapy. In chapter seven, we discussed less extreme cases where a manipulative or deceptive intervention is used to jolt a patient out of an entrenched pattern of heteronomy. One needs to interpret the principle and to allow for exceptions in extreme cases. But if there are to be exceptions in extreme cases, how extreme do the cases have to be, and how are they to be identified? It is difficult to see how such questions could be answered within a tolerably short code of ethics.

Confidentiality is thought to be essential to the therapeutic relationship, and there are good reasons for supposing that therapists have the strongest obligation not to divulge what has been revealed to them in therapy. Moreover, without a strong expectation of confidentiality it is likely that many would-be patients would avoid therapy and be denied its benefits, and that those within therapy would be inhibited in what they said. This would seriously undermine the therapeutic process. In this case, unlike the others, there is no problem of interpretation. However, difficulties remain because, on reflection, there are compelling reasons for allowing some exceptions to the "no breach of confidence" rule. The most obvious case is where the therapist believes, on the basis of information provided by a patient, that there is a serious risk of the patient committing murder or suicide. This situation is, in important respects, analogous to that where it is legitimate to deceive.

There is good reason to include the prohibition on psychotherapy being used as a form of social control, because there are fears that the considerable power that therapists may have over their patients could be used to impose social conformity on patients or prisoners judged to be deviant. Without such a prohibition, patients may be abused and individual therapists placed in an invidiously compromising position. Once again, however, there is a serious difficulty of interpretation. Consider our example from chapter eight, of family therapy being used with a school-refusing teenager as an alternative to the teenager being placed in care. On the one hand, the therapy might be seen as a way of producing social conformity in the child and her family; on the other, it may be less controlling and less coercive than the likely alternative remedies to the child's social problems. Similar difficulties are raised by the use of behaviour therapy in prisons.

One conclusion that we draw from these considerations is that a code of psychotherapeutic ethics, whatever else it might do, is unlikely to remove the need for therapists to use their individual judgement in the solution of the moral dilemmas that will confront them from time to time in their work. The moral problems that are likely to occur in therapy are too complicated to be resolved by a simple set of principles. In so far as potential patients need protection from the dangers of abuse by therapists, it is unlikely that a brief code of ethics based along the line of the International Code of Medical Ethics would go far in helping to provide it.

One way for professional bodies to try to make good these deficiencies in their codes of ethics is to offer detailed interpretations of the clauses in the codes. This is useful, although the interpretations are inevitably far longer than the original codes. A good example is the American Medical Association's *Principles of Medical Ethics with Annotations Especially Applicable to Psychiatry* (American Psychiatric Association, 1985). The Foreword to this annotated statement of the principles states:

> While psychiatrists have the same goals as all physicians, there are special ethical problems in psychiatric practice that differ in colouring and degree from ethical problems in other branches of medical practice, even though the basic principles are the same.

> The annotations are not designed as absolutes and will be re-
> vised from time to time so as to be applicable to current practices
> and problems. [American Psychiatric Association, 1985]

The annotations go far beyond the initial general statements; they include specific directives for particular dilemmas and even mention sanctions to be adopted against offending psychiatrists. The simple principle "A physician shall respect the rights of patients, colleagues, and of other health professionals, and shall safeguard patient confidences within the constraints of the law" is given thirteen paragraphs of notes, including statements as specific as:

> Ethically the psychiatrist may disclose only that information
> which is relevant to a given situation. He/she should avoid offer-
> ing speculation as fact. Sensitive information such as an individu-
> al's sexual orientation or fantasy material is usually unnecessary.
> [American Psychiatric Association, 1985]

With the annotations, the principles have effectively become a *code of practice*, which we believe would be of far greater value for psychotherapy than a more general or abstract code of ethics.

Codes of ethics and codes of practice

Suppose a company, on moral grounds, wishes to stamp out racism and sexism in appointments made by its managers. It could, as part of a code of ethics, decree that sexism and racism in appointments, being unethical, are unacceptable in the company. This worthy state-ment of principle is unlikely to be effective without the back-up of a *code of practice*. A code of practice is really a set of detailed statements setting out how broadly defined policy objectives are to be imple-mented. In the case of the employer who wants to eliminate racism and sexism from appointment decisions, it might include something like the following, which is taken from Bradford Metropolitan Dis-trict Council's Code of Practice for recruitment and selection (City of Bradford Metropolitan District Council, 1985):

> A written personnel specification must be produced for every
> vacancy. It must focus entirely on the qualifications and experi-
> ence that are needed for the job. The personnel specification must
> NOT specify that a recruit will be of a particular SEX, ETHNIC
> ORIGIN, or RELIGION. The personnel specification must NOT

specify that a recruit will be MARRIED, or SINGLE, or HAVE
PARTICULAR HOME CIRCUMSTANCES (such as having no
children). The reasons for appointing a recruit must refer to the
personnel specification alone.

A code of practice usually contains not only mandatory requirements such as those above, failure to comply with which may result
in disciplinary proceedings, but also a set of recommendations about
good practice which, perhaps because they are too complex to be
implemented by simple instructions, are not mandatory. Here is an
example of the latter, again taken from Bradford's Code of Practice:

> Unless we have a clear idea of the qualities we are looking for,
> and a clear idea of how to assess them—we will tend to choose
> people we feel comfortable with. Usually that means people
> from a similar background, and with a similar, traditional educa-
> tion, to ourselves. ... Similarly, if we are not concentrating on
> getting hard evidence about a candidate's abilities, we may also
> tend to concentrate on irrelevancies such as "the impression they
> made on me" or "how they could fit into the office." We should
> ask ourselves hard questions about these: Are we paying people
> to make a good impression on me? Are we paying them to fit into
> a happy office? How do we know who will "fit into an office"?

It is not our concern to discuss the merits of Bradford's Code of
Practice, but simply to use these extracts to illustrate our point. A
code of practice can include well-defined requirements that can be
enforced by an employer or a professional body. They can also include recommendations for good practice.

Within psychotherapy, as our discussion in chapter four reveals,
there is a particular need to eliminate subtle forms of unwarranted
discrimination. There is also a need for guidelines to determine, for
example, when it is acceptable for a therapist to breach a confidence
and, if so, how it should be done; to decide whether sexual contact
between therapist and patient is ever to be tolerated; to place limits
on the use of behaviour therapy in prisons; and so on. It seems to us
that, although a specific code of psychotherapeutic ethics is unlikely
to be of much use, there is a compelling case for a code of practice for
psychotherapy. Such a code might be contained in a handbook that
would be given to all psychotherapy students and practitioners,
and would properly be produced by a professional psychotherapy
council such as the UKCP. It could also be made available to patients,

perhaps by being displayed in therapists' waiting rooms. Most psychotherapy organizations have their own codes of ethics, and some have their own code of practice. What we are proposing is a code of ethical practice for psychotherapists as a group, which would become part of a recognized professional practice.

It would be presumptuous of us to attempt to produce a sample code—and anyway it would take us beyond the scope of this book. One thing is clear, however. If there is to be an effective code of practice for *psychotherapists*, there will have to be bodies responsible for drawing up and revising such a code, and for enforcing adherence to it. This, we believe, is part of the task of the psychotherapy profession. In the next chapter, we develop the case for a psychotherapy profession, describing—and we hope answering—the major objections to it.

CHAPTER TEN

Psychotherapy:
the makings of a profession

Despite a long history (Ellenberger, 1970) and considerable cultural significance, the status of psychotherapy remains ambiguous. Many who practise psychotherapy are members of established professions—psychiatrists, psychologists, social workers. Psychoanalysis claims to be a profession but was described by Freud, in a moment of ambivalence, as an "impossible" one—"because one can be sure beforehand of reaching unsatisfying results" (Freud, 1937c). But psychotherapy ranges from its conventional and established centre to obscure and quasi-religious fringes. Despite aspirations to acceptance and respectability, psychotherapy as a whole does not yet present the public with the unity and ideological coherence that are the hallmarks of a profession.

It should also be noted that within psychotherapy there are those for whom the very notion of respectability is contradictory. They see the subversiveness and ramshackle aspect of psychotherapy as a necessary consequence of the radical nature of its subject-matter. If psychotherapy is to confront (and be trusted by) that which is repressed, how can it ally itself with the very forces of convention and normality which are responsible for that repression? "Psychoanalysis is like a nomadic tribe, never settling in any one place" (Kohon, 1984).

We have, to some extent, discussed this issue in chapter five and will not pursue it further here, except to note that the ambivalence that it represents has probably played no small part in the slow progress that psychotherapy has made towards achieving professional status.

In this chapter, we consider some of the obstacles that need to be overcome if, as we believe it should, psychotherapy is to become an established profession. This claim, which has been developed throughout this book, is based on the argument that without a broad and united psychotherapy profession it will be virtually impossible to guarantee the standards of training and ethics that are needed if psychotherapy is properly to serve the public.

In the first part of the book we argued that psychotherapy can be an effective way of alleviating mental distress, including some forms of psychiatric illness. We claimed that its distinctive contribution derives from its focus on the enhancement of emotional autonomy and of the capacity to form satisfying relationships, and that these benefits are essential to the well-being of a wide range of people with a variety of difficulties. We then emphasized how, although there is a strong case for psychotherapy to be recognized as a part of essential care, it is in very short supply: large sections of the population are denied access to skilled psychotherapy, because of geography, class, education, or income. We suggested that this discrepancy between need and availability could be overcome by a significant expansion of appropriate state-funded psychotherapy, and that the likely benefits of this provision by the state far outweigh the possible dangers.

But if the public funds spent on psychotherapy are to be greatly expanded, then the taxpayer and potential patients will rightly demand that psychotherapists are technically competent. This will depend on organized training and monitoring, and the best way to ensure this is for psychotherapists to organize themselves as a profession.

Our second main argument for the development of a psychotherapy profession springs directly from the ethical problems that arise within psychotherapy. We have shown how the different modes and contexts of use of psychotherapy create their own special ethical problems and that these make psychotherapy liable to particular forms of abuse.

The need for a profession to set and maintain ethical standards was very clearly stated in Sir John Foster's Report to the British government, published in 1971:

It is high time that the practice of psychotherapy for reward should be restricted to members of a profession properly qualified in its techniques and trained—as all organised professions are trained—to use the patient's dependence which flows from the inherent inequality of the relationship only for the good of the patient himself, and never for the exploitation of his weakness to the therapist's profit. [Foster, 1971]

Sir John recommended that:

Psychotherapy (in the general sense of the treatment for fee or reward of illnesses, complaints, or problems, by psychological means) should be organised as a restricted profession open only to those who undergo an appropriate training and are willing to adhere to a . . . proper code of ethics, and . . . the necessary legislation should be drafted and presented to Parliament as soon as possible. [Foster, 1971]

We can see clearly some of the difficulties of establishing a psychotherapy profession if we consider the experience in Britain following the Foster Report. In 1971, it looked as if psychotherapy in Britain was, on the basis of Foster, set fair to become a profession. In 1975, at the suggestion of the Department of Health and Social Security (DHSS), a joint working party was set up consisting of representatives from interested parties (including the British Psycho-Analytic Society, the British Association of Behavioural Psychotherapy, the Royal College of Psychiatrists, and the DHSS) under the chairmanship of a lawyer from Sir John's Chambers, the late Mr Paul Sieghart. The Working Party produced a report, known as the "Sieghart Report" (Sieghart, 1979), recommending:

1. statutory regulation of psychotherapists;

2. the formation of a statutory body called the Council for Psychotherapy; and

3. the establishment of an inspectorate of training courses.

However, by the 1980s, the situation had changed. The original Joint Working Party included representatives both from *established* professions such as the Royal College of Psychiatrists (1983) and the Joint Board of Clinical Nursing, and from psychotherapy organizations *aspiring* to professional recognition, such as the British Association of

Psychotherapists. Collaboration began to break down. The "core professions", comprising psychiatry, social work, psychology, and nursing, were becoming less enthusiastic about an independent psychotherapy profession. This was especially true of psychology and nursing, which, as relatively new professions themselves, were more concerned about their own claims to autonomy and status. The British Psychological Society argued that state-funded psychotherapy should be provided only by *already established* professions such as psychology. Meanwhile, in the years between 1971 and 1981, many independent psychotherapy training organizations had established themselves, including Institutes of Family Therapy, Humanistic Psychotherapy, and Behaviour Therapy. All sought recognition and wanted to be included in the process of setting up a psychotherapy profession. They were viewed with some suspicion by the older psychotherapy organizations, especially the psychoanalysts. There followed two sets of "status wars"—firstly between the established professions and the psychotherapists, and secondly among the different psychotherapy organizations themselves. Consensus had, at least temporarily, broken down. But without consensus, the Government argued, no Bill other than a Private Member's Bill with a negligible chance of reaching the Statute Book, could be introduced.

With the DHSS and the Government pulling back from the idea of a register of professionally accredited psychotherapists (the key to state recognition of the profession), the onus fell on psychotherapists to put their house in order. This led to the establishment of annual meetings of the United Kingdom Standing Conference for Psychotherapy, the so-called "Rugby" conferences (named after the venue of the first meeting), which brought together psychotherapy organizations interested in creating a psychotherapy profession and led to the drawing up of training standards and ethical guidelines. At the inaugural meeting in 1982, there were thirty member organizations; by 1989 the membership had increased to over seventy. In 1993 a register of psychotherapists was established under the auspices of the newly formed United Kingdom Council for Psychotherapy (UKCP). UKCP has a federal structure in which psychotherapy training organizations are grouped together according to their orientation or stance— for example, psychoanalytic, behavioural, family and marital, humanistic, university courses in psychotherapy, and so on. Individual practitioners are registered via their parent organization. The role of UKCP is to set standards for training and ethical conduct for member organizations, of which there are currently around eighty.

The establishment of UKCP was a great leap forward in the path towards recognition as a profession, but major difficulties remain. A group of analytically oriented organizations have split away from UKCP to form their own umbrella body, the British Confederation of Psychotherapists (BCP). The BCP, along with a number of other organizations, are publishing their own register of psychotherapists. Government continues to maintain a hands-off position about statutory recognition, perhaps seeing psychotherapists as too riven with internecine struggles to speak with a common voice. It has, however, published a seminal report surveying the state of psychotherapy within the NHS, which calls for a much stronger psychotherapy presence within psychiatry and medicine (NHSE, 1996).

What, then, are the remaining issues that need to be settled if psychotherapy is to become a profession? Are there any serious disadvantages of psychotherapy becoming a profession? If professionalization does take place, how should psychotherapists organize and deploy themselves?

Professions and their disadvantages

According to Talcott Parsons (Parsons, 1951), a key feature of professions is their "collectivity orientation". By this he means that the ideology and overt aim of professions is improved public welfare, rather than personal or sectional selfishness. In his view, when a novitiate joins a profession she gives up some individuality and takes on the "higher" standards and norms of the profession as a whole. Her aim becomes that of service, rather than self-seeking. Similarly, the profession as a whole, rather than attempting to maximize sales and profit as do commercial organizations, aims to meet public need. Parsons was wrestling with the problems of how social care could coexist with a fiercely capitalist system like that in the United States. But this optimistic view of professions is by no means universally shared. Bernard Shaw saw professions as "conspiracies against the laity", and Ivan Illich has campaigned against the professions, which, in his view, far from serving the public, create dependency and, in the case of medicine, disease, by an iatrogenesis that produces results far more damaging than any microbe (Illich, 1975).

Consider the following list of "traits" compiled by the sociologist William Goode, distinguishing "professions" from the "occupations" out of which they have emerged:

(1) The profession determines its own standards of education and training.

(2) The student professional goes through a more far-reaching adult socialization experience than the learner in other occupations.

(3) Professional practice is often legally recognized by some form of licensure.

(4) Licensing and admission boards are manned by members of the profession.

(5) Most legislation concerned with the profession is shaped by the profession.

(6) The occupation gains in income, power, and prestige ranking, and can demand higher calibre students.

(7) The practitioner is relatively free of lay evaluation and control.

(8) The norms of practice enforced by the profession are more stringent than legal controls.

(9) Members are more strongly identified and affiliated with the profession than are members of other occupations with theirs.

(10) The profession is more likely to be a terminal occupation [sic]. Members do not care to leave it, and a higher proportion assert that if they had it to do over again, they would again choose that type of work. [Goode, 1960]

The list is far from homogeneous. It includes both features genuinely likely to enhance quality of service and protect the public from abuse, such as regulation of training and norms of practice, and those concerned with professional self-interest, like enhanced prestige and freedom from lay control.

The professionalization of psychotherapy would, on the whole, we believe, be in the public interest. But the heterogeneity of Goode's list reminds us that there is no *guarantee* that this would be so. Even if professionalization were to raise standards and set acceptable ethical norms, it might also lead, for example, to esotericism and protectionism. These dangers must be borne in mind alongside the undoubted advantages that a psychotherapy profession would bring.

We now consider in some detail a number of the specific problems that must be solved before the professionalization of psychotherapy can come about. There are two main issues: a conceptual problem about how to decide what is and what is not to be included within "psychotherapy"; and a *practical* problem—how to unite the many factions, tendencies, and groupings that all practise or claim to practise psychotherapy.

The boundaries of psychotherapy

The full title of Foster's Report, from which we have quoted, was: *An Enquiry into the Practice and Effects of Scientology*. The enquiry was set up because of a public outcry about the "abduction and corruption" of vulnerable young people by L. Ron Hubbard's Church of Scientology, which described scientology itself as "the first thoroughly validated psychotherapy". Foster argued that if scientology were to be outlawed, and thereby distinguished from reputable psychotherapy, it would be necessary for psychotherapy itself to move towards professional status and to accept statutory regulation of its activities.

The existence of a profession implies a *boundary* that separates it from other professions and from non-professional activities. The act of professing is the gateway across that boundary and usually includes rites of passage such as the passing of exams or other guarantees of having successfully completed work preparatory to entry. The term "profession" derives from the declaration or vow taken by novitiates on entering a religious order. The effect of a boundary is, by definition, divisive. "Insiders" and "outsiders" are created, as Foster implied in his Report.

If psychotherapy is to become a profession, where should the boundary be drawn and by whom, and how should it be enforced? A liberal boundary would admit some undesirable practices and practitioners, but could encourage innovation and variety. A restrictive boundary, on the other hand, would ensure standards but could stifle change and exclude potentially good therapists. Boundaries inevitably affect vested interests. New professions like psychotherapy encroach on older ones like psychology and psychiatry. Newer therapies like family therapy challenge established ones like psycho-analysis, and professionals in general may have a vested interest in discouraging self-help by the public.

In the establishment of the medical profession, one of the main factors that held up what was to become the 1858 Medical Registration Act was the question of "quacks". When eventually the Act was passed, one of its main functions was to create a register of officially recognized medical practitioners. There were about 15,000, of whom 10,000 were qualified practitioners but 5,000 were "quacks", unqualified doctors achieving licensure through custom rather than qualification (Sieghart, 1979).

For a similar unified register of psychotherapists to be created, serious boundary questions would have to be settled. First, if a register of official psychotherapists is created, what about all the unofficial psychotherapy that goes on, say, between teachers and pupils, priests and parishioners, or even palmists and their "palmisands"? Should this be automatically outlawed?

Second, what should happen to professionals in disciplines related to psychotherapy, such as medicine, social work, or psychology? Should they be automatically included within the boundary of psychotherapy, even though their training in formal psychotherapy may be very superficial?

Third, what about the differences between psychotherapy trainings, which vary greatly in length, breadth, and depth? Should they all be considered equal when it comes to the registration of psychotherapists and the accreditation of psychotherapy training schemes?

One hallmark of a profession is that its practitioners have technical knowledge and skill that do not exist, or exist in only a rudimentary form, outside the profession. This creates a problem for psychotherapists whose skills, being to do with people rather than things, and with people as people, rather than people as things, can be hard to specify as compared, for example, with those of an architect or a chiropodist. This difficulty had led some to respond to boundary questions by denying the distinction between psychotherapy and other helping professions. They resist the idea that there are any particular skills or training needed to practise psychotherapy. This defensive response is particularly prevalent among non-psychotherapist psychiatrists, who argue that since psychotherapy is about talking to people, and since psychiatrists talk to their patients, it follows that "we are all psychotherapists now", and there is no need for a special profession to be created. This is no less absurd than arguing that since everyone removes splinters from time to time there is no need for specially trained surgeons, or, to make an oedipal analogy, that since parents can love both their children and their spouses there are no differences between conjugal and parental love. It blurs the important distinction between informal and formal psychotherapy.

At the opposite extreme, some hold that only formal psychotherapy, or often some particular version of it such as psychoanalysis, is real psychotherapy, and that the public must be protected at all costs from attenuated or watered-down versions that masquerade as the real thing. One problem with this position is that it ossifies the existing structure of psychotherapy and may inhibit the development of new theories and practices. Moreover, it fails to recognize that, as we argued in chapter four, "watered-down" psychotherapy may at times be exactly what some people need. Watering down has legitimate as well as perverse purposes. An edict insisting that French children must no longer drink watered-down wine at family meals would lead either to a lot more drunk children, or to much less well-socialized ones.

The Sieghart solution

How, then, can psychotherapy define a boundary that is both broad enough to include the range and variety of psychotherapies, and yet narrow enough to exclude charlatans? This was the question that Sieghart's Working Party set itself (Sieghart, 1979). Their solution was ingenious. It turned on the distinction between *functional* and *indicative* registration. In some professions, it is illegal for a non-registered individual to practise. A non-registered medical doctor who performs an operation may be guilty of battery. The register of medical practitioners both *indicates* those who have passed the relevant examinations and have maintained a proper standard of professional conduct, and specifies *the functions* that doctors *are* trained and licensed to perform. Such a *functional* register would, Sieghart argued, be inappropriate for psychotherapy, since the types of psychotherapeutic activity are so varied. A functional definition of what psychotherapists should be allowed to do would exclude many valuable informal psychotherapeutic activities such as counselling by teachers, priests, or social workers. But some setting of boundaries is needed if the public is to be protected by legislation from unqualified practitioners.

Sieghart therefore proposed *indicative* registration for psychotherapy. This protects the *title* of psychotherapist, but not the activity of psychotherapy (being psychotherapeutic). Anyone may design their own house or tend to a sick relative, but only those who have received an approved training may call themselves architects or nurses. If indicative registration were adopted, only those who received a recognized training would be entitled to *call* themselves psychotherapists, although anyone would remain free to "psychotherapize".

Freud, "lay" analysis, and quackery

The aim of the Sieghart proposals was to exclude psychotherapeutic quackery without denying the importance of informal psychotherapy. Of course, not all problems would be solved by a Sieghart-type indicative register. An unregistered psychotherapist would only have to change her title to, say, "psycho-integrationist", in order to continue to practise quite legally. A more serious boundary question that the Seighart proposals fail to solve concerns the relationship between the established "core professions" of medicine, nursing, social work, and psychology, and a new profession of psychotherapy.

It is interesting at this point to consider an analogous problem that arose early in the history of the psychoanalytic movement. In 1926, T. Reik, a non-medical but highly scrupulous (see chapter seven) psychoanalyst practising in Vienna, was charged, under an old Austrian law that prohibited non-medical people from treating patients, with "quackery". This led to an argument within the psychoanalytic movement about the position of non-medical ("lay") analysts. Some, particularly the American psychoanalysts, argued that *all* analysts should be medically qualified. Others, Freud included, argued with equal force in favour of lay analysis. Two issues that emerged in this debate are of immediate contemporary relevance: first, the attitude of an older profession to a new one, and

second, the role of legislation in regulating the activities of psychotherapists.

In contrast to the American analysts, Freud argued that the qualifications necessary to practise psychotherapy were not those legal
requirements imposed by a state that had no knowledge of the
subject (British Government departmental publications regularly
confuse psychotherapy with physiotherapy!), but genuine understanding of the subject and relevant training. He was as much
opposed to doctors unqualified in psychotherapy practising it, as
he was to so-called "quacks":

> Permit me to give the word "quack" the meaning it ought to have
> instead of the legal one. According to the law, a quack is anyone
> who treats patients without possessing a state diploma to prove
> he is a doctor. I should prefer another definition: a quack is
> anyone who undertakes a treatment without possessing the
> knowledge and capacities necessary for it. Taking my stand on
> this definition, I venture to assert that—not only in European
> countries—doctors form a preponderating contingent of quacks
> in analysis. They very frequently practise analytic treatment
> without having learnt it and without understanding it. [Freud,
> 1926e]

Despite being critical of doctors untrained in psychotherapy offering
"psychoanalysis", Freud was opposed to prohibitive legislation for
similar baby-and-bathwater reasons to those for which Seighart rejected the compulsory functional registration of psychotherapists: he
feared that a strict law might exclude lay analysts, whose cause he
passionately championed, along with the medical "pseudo-analysts"
whom he criticized. His libertarian view is revealed in the following
passage:

> Let us allow patients themselves to discover that it is damaging
> to them to look for mental assistance to people who have not
> learnt how to give it. If we explain this to them and warn them
> against it, we shall have spared ourselves the need to forbid it.
> On the main roads of Italy the pylons that carry high-tension
> cables bear the brief and impressive inscription: "Chi tocca,
> muore" ("He who touches will die"). This is perfectly calculated
> to regulate the behaviour of passers-by to any wires that may
> be hanging down. The corresponding German notices exhibit
> an unnecessary and offensive verbosity: "Das Beruhren der

Leitungsdrahte ist, weil lebensgefahrlich, strengsten verboten" ("Touching the cables is, since it is dangerous to life, most strictly prohibited"). Why the prohibition? Anyone who holds his life dear will make the prohibition for himself; and anyone who wants to kill himself in that way will not ask for permission. [Freud, 1926e]

Freud, faced with a choice between functional registration and none at all, opted for none at all. Sieghart's proposed indicative registration, which protects the title but not the function, provides a useful third way that is neither too permissive nor too restrictive.

Psychoanalysts, following Freud's lead, initially took a neutral attitude towards the formation of a psychotherapy profession. One reason for this is that psychoanalysis, although (at least in some countries) affording full and equal status to non-medical analysts, has always been strongly allied to medicine, with many of its pre-eminent members being medically qualified. Many psychoanalysts achieve status and recognition through medicine rather than as psychotherapists, and so they are not strongly motivated either to support or to oppose a new psychotherapy profession.

The situation is very different for the new core professions of clinical psychology, nursing, and social work, all of which have had and are still having to fight hard against psychiatric resistance to "encroachment". They are striving to establish themselves as valid professions, and, perhaps not surprisingly, it is now clinical psychologists who are among the most opposed to the establishment of a new profession of psychotherapy.

Psychotherapy and the core professions

In our view, this opposition, while understandable, is difficult to defend. There are powerful arguments in favour of psychotherapy's bid to become a new profession overlapping with, but separate from, general medicine, psychiatry, nursing, clinical psychology, and social work.

First, it is in the nature of psychotherapy that none of the existing professions can legitimately claim a monopoly on it. Psychoanalysts are trained in psychoanalysis, but only a minority of patients in need of psychotherapy will benefit from full psychoanalysis. Clinical psychologists may have special training and expertise in cognitive behavioural therapies but have little knowledge, training, or interest in psychodynamic therapies. Psychiatrists may have extensive training in psychotherapy, or almost none. The older professions, due to their sectional interests, are unlikely to achieve either the breadth of training or the depth of funding required to meet the overall demand for psychotherapy in the population.

Second, for the core professions, formal psychotherapy, as opposed to informal psychotherapy, is only a *part*—and sometimes only a small part—of what they do: psychiatrists prescribe drugs, clinical psychologists test IQs and give vocational advice, social workers arrange housing for their clients. None of these is central to the psychotherapist's brief.

Third, when members of the core professions undertake special training in psychotherapy, they enter a new professional mode and role and, to a large extent, leave their previous profession behind. When doing psychotherapy, psychiatrists, psychologists, social workers, and lay therapists are, on the whole, indistinguishable. They are defined by being psychotherapists rather than by the profession from which they came. As a result, therapists from different backgrounds will be found doing the same job, but under very different pay and conditions. This is neither efficient nor equitable.

Fourth, without a distinct profession of psychotherapy the needs of the population for psychotherapy are likely to be met only piecemeal, and by therapists who lack the necessary training and knowledge of the range of therapies.

A fifth argument for a psychotherapy profession, encompassing but distinct from the core professions, with its own entry requirements and training, is that, as Freud recognized, psychotherapy is, or can be, a "calling" in its own right. If psychotherapists were restricted to members of one of the core professions, many potentially good therapists (for example, with an "Arts" background) might be discouraged, either because they lacked the necessary formal qualifications or because, rightly, they would see this preliminary training as an unnecessary and expensive diversion from their chosen course.

In this section, we have supported Sieghart's original proposals for an indicative register of psychotherapists, now a central part of the work of the UKCP. A register promotes the improved standards of training and practice which are needed if psychotherapy is to become part of essential care. Indicative registration could mean, for instance, that only *registered* psychotherapists could be employed in publicly funded posts, or be paid for under publicly funded insurance schemes. It is worth stressing that this move would, to some extent, be a threat to existing professions, and that it almost directly contradicts the views of the British Psychological Society, which has argued that registration of psychotherapists is necessary only for the *private* sector, while state-funded therapists should all be members of a recognized profession such as psychology or social work. This, we believe, misses the point that psychotherapy has a separate and special contribution to make within a state-funded service, and that the training needed for this, while overlapping to some extent with that undergone by other professions, is unique.

We are encouraged that the NHS Psychotherapy Review (NHSE, 1996) comes to similar conclusions. The review distinguishes between three types of psychotherapy delivery: (A) psychotherapy as part of general psychiatric management (for example, family therapy as part of the treatment of schizophrenia), (B) eclectic client-oriented therapies, often delivered by clinical psychologists based in community mental health teams, and (C) formal psychotherapies such as CBT and analytic therapy, often delivered by psychotherapy departments to patients with complex and difficult problems. Type C psychotherapy depends on the existence of a distinct profession of psychotherapy with its own professional training and standards. The review argues that this is the best guarantee that appropriate, "evidence-based" treatments will be offered in an ethical way to potential clients.

Unity and diversity in psychotherapy

In the early 1800s, barber surgeons, smart Harley Street physicians, lithotomists, and workhouse doctors would hardly have considered themselves members of a common profession. Yet, little more than half a century later, they were beginning to bed down together under the Medical Registration Act of 1858 (General Medical Council, 1958).

The establishment of a professional register of psychotherapists under government statute would bring together a very diverse group of practitioners. There are at present many strata among psychotherapists, and this is partly reflected in the training required for different kinds of therapy. Psychoanalysts and analytical psychologists undergo the most intensive and prolonged training. As direct disciples or descendants of Freud or Jung, they lay claim to the true ark of the covenant of the unconscious. Family therapists can claim more social relevance and general applicability than analysts. Behaviour therapists, whose training is much briefer but on the whole available only to established professionals like nurses and psychologists, claim statistical and scientific validation for their methods that other therapies lack. Newer organizations like the British Association of Psychotherapists base their training closely on a briefer version of the psychoanalytic model. The newer "humanistic" expressive therapies claim immediate access to the unconscious and often more varied and less intellectually demanding trainings.

The new therapists tend to find psychoanalysts stuffy and conventional: analysts view these "upstart arrivals" with suspicion, or even disdain. But, as we have argued repeatedly throughout the book, only a *diversity* of psychotherapies can meet the overall need of the population for psychotherapeutic treatment. The task facing those wishing to create a profession of psychotherapy is to weld these very disparate groups into a common whole. To succeed as a profession, this unity has to be more than just a temporary coincidence of interest.

In any profession there is a need for a common philosophy and shared basic assumptions about the relevant sphere of knowledge. In some ways, psychotherapy would appear to be an exception to this rule. Unlike conventional medicine, where all practitioners are concerned with the same basic anatomy, physiology, and biochemistry, psychotherapy is about those aspects of people which make them individual, unique, and diverse. The variety of psychotherapy schools and trainings is therefore inherent in the nature of the discipline. The variety of people and the differences between their needs mean that psychotherapies will inevitably continue to be varied, even after the formation of a profession. Any exclusive claim on psychotherapeutic primacy or truth should be regarded with great suspicion.

Nor can unity be achieved by a naive eclecticism. Good psychotherapy is not a stew in which the best of all the different ingredients for human growth can be blended. The different therapies need to retain their identity while working in a more united and collaborative way. As suggested in chapter two, eclecticism in psychotherapy is useful when it means that therapists with different approaches come to see what they have in common—the cognitive features of psychoanalysis, the transferential aspects of behaviour therapy—but not as an amalgam of incompatible elements.

A psychotherapy profession would be an arena in which this collaboration could be fostered for the benefit of the public. It would also help to overcome a real difficulty that exists for the consumer faced with the variety of psychotherapies. Most psychotherapists are specialists only in their own particular branch of therapy. The person in search of help is faced with an array of different treatments and is often not in a position or state to evaluate the distinctions between them and so make an informed choice of therapy. Therapists them-selves are at present little better off. Psychoanalysts may have little knowledge of or interest in the indications for and benefits of behav-iour therapy, and *vice versa*. There is an understandable tendency for therapists to assume that their own approach is *the* one that can help the patient. A psychotherapy profession is needed if the cacophony of one-man bands is to be harmonized for the benefit of the would-be patient.

A psychotherapy council: essential forum or self-serving bureaucracy?

There is an argument that holds that the establishment of a psycho-therapy bureaucracy, and all the paraphernalia of professionalism, are inimical to the spirit of psychotherapy. We have argued up to this point in favour of professionalization, especially when psycho-therapy is delivered through a state-funded organization such as the NHS. How, in practice, can organizations such as the UKCP prove their worth? Registers of psychotherapists have now been estab-lished. The UKCP has a federal psychotherapy council in which the different psychotherapeutic disciplines are represented under a com-mon umbrella organization. What has the UKCP achieved so far? A key task has been to set up an ethics committee to establish codes of practice for psychotherapists. A second essential role has been the supervision and accreditation of training schemes (Pedder, 1988). We would argue that another important job is to seek proper funding for psychotherapy, as well as to ensure an equitable distribution of such resources as already exist. We argued earlier in favour of conceiving of psychotherapy in the broadest terms, and that people's essential need for enhanced emotional autonomy and satisfying personal relationships requires a wide deployment of psychotherapists and a significant use of state funding.

An ethics committee and codes of practice for psychotherapists

In the previous four chapters, we discussed some of the ethical issues that arise within psychotherapy. Some of these questions arise for all therapists, such as what to do when therapist and patient are tempted to start a sexual relationship, how to handle complaints arising from possible "false memories", and how to balance patient "consumer sovereignty" against the need for protection from extortionate or interminable therapy. Others are specific to particular forms of treatment, like the issue of self-revelation in analytic therapy, or negative reinforcement schedules in behaviour therapy, or manipulation in family therapy.

Ethical issues like these shade off in two very different directions. One is in the direction of discipline for practitioners who transgress ethical guidelines. For instance, an ethics committee has to decide what should be done about practitioners who are alleged to be abusing their position by having sexual relationships with patients. How are such cases to be heard? If guilty, should therapists lose their registration? If so, for how long? Ethical questions lead in this direction to issues of boundaries and ultimately to who is or is not fit to be a member of the psychotherapy profession.

At the same time, ethical questions also lead away from the boundaries into everyday practice. There is need to find arrangements for psychotherapy that will make it less, rather than more, likely that serious offences will occur, and to improve the general tenor and atmosphere within which psychotherapy is practised.

Specific questions are likely to arise within individual training organizations. What rules of confidentiality do and should apply within a particular psychotherapy department? Are potential psychotherapy patients being offered comprehensive assessment interviews and the possibility of treatment across the range of psychotherapies? Are cases reviewed for progress at regular intervals, with appropriate letters to referrers such as GPs? Do all practitioners have access to supervision? How much choice of therapist or therapy do patients get when they enter treatment? How much effort is made to reach disadvantaged groups who may benefit from, but have little access to, psychotherapy? These questions need to be asked, and should be carefully considered, if a psychotherapy service really is to become more equitable.

So an ethics committee has two main functions: first, to establish disciplinary procedures for "policing" a register of psychotherapists; second, to produce codes of practice, both general and specific to the various forms of psychotherapy, and find ways of monitoring how different psychotherapists, psychotherapy group practices, and psychotherapy departments apply these codes. As argued in chapter nine, we are, on the whole, sceptical about the efficacy or relevance of exhortatory codes of ethics issued *ex cathedra* by a governing council. Only detailed, time-consuming, and potentially costly work in preparing, evaluating, and enforcing codes of practice is likely to have a significant impact on the day-to-day practice of psychotherapy in a way that will benefit the public.

Selection, training, and accreditation

One of the main benefits to the public of the current moves towards establishing a statutory profession of psychotherapy has been the focus on professional training standards. Remuneration in state-funded psychotherapy schemes such as NHS psychotherapy departments could be confined to registered psychotherapists, all of whom would have been trained on a programme accredited by the psychotherapy council.

The psychotherapy council has to consider two main questions related to training: who should be accepted for psychotherapy training, and what should be the structure and content of their courses? Most current psychotherapy trainings lay down certain essential requirements for candidates: a minimum age (for example, 25), some experience in the field of care or counselling, and a university degree. Many trainings attempt to assess the candidate's maturity and balance, and to exclude those who are drawn to psychotherapy because of their own psychological disturbance, rather than a genuine vocation. These are very delicate matters, and again it is difficult to set standards that are neither too permissive nor too strict. As James Glover said in 1925: "The most pessimistic criticism of psychotherapy I have ever heard was the opinion that no one ought to practise psychotherapy unless he had the wisdom of Socrates and the morality of Jesus Christ" (quoted in Halmos, 1965).

There is a danger that a psychotherapy profession could create a bureaucracy that would exclude potentially creative or unusual candidates. James Strachey, who became a prominent psychoanalyst and the official translator of Freud, graphically expressed the danger when he compared the application forms and required curriculae vitarum of the established Psycho-Analytic Society of the 1960s with his own experience in the 1920s:

> Documents of this kind fill me with bloodcurdling feelings of anxiety and remorse. How on earth could I fill up one of them? A discreditable academic career with the barest of BA degrees, no medical qualifications, no knowledge of the physical sciences, no experience of anything except third-rate journalism. The only thing in my favour was that, at the age of thirty, I wrote a letter to Freud, asking him if he would take me on as a student. For some reason he replied, almost by return of post, that he would. . . . Whether it is possible for it to become over-institutionalized is an open question. Is it worthwhile to leave a loophole for an occasional maverick? [quoted in Kohon, 1986]

A psychotherapy council should look critically at the way training courses select candidates. There are, as we have seen, two kinds of error that training organizations can fall into: being too liberal, thereby selecting unsuitable candidates, and being too rigid, thereby excluding or putting off many potential good therapists. One role of the council would be to minimize the risks of these kinds of errors being made.

There is fairly widespread agreement that any adequate training in psychotherapy will include the three components *theory, supervised practice,* and *some element of personal development or therapy,* although strict behaviourists might object to the last. We would argue that the special ethical difficulties associated with psychotherapy make it particularly important that some form of moral development is incorporated within any psychotherapy training. Psychotherapists cannot be Christ- or Socrates-like, but they do need to develop a special ethical sensitivity, including an awareness of their own fallibility, if they are to cope with the demands of their work and avoid falling into the traps that we have discussed in previous chapters. Personal therapy is one way to achieve this. The psychotherapy council would be concerned not just with ethical guidelines and discipline, but also with how psychotherapy trainings can help foster their candidates' personal and ethical development. Whether a candidate in a training organization "passes" or "fails" appears at present an arbitrary decision of a training committee. We believe that there is a need for trainings to become much more open in their teaching methods generally and, in particular, to make explicit the criteria by which academic, technical, and personal competence are judged. When candidates are "failed", as inevitably a proportion will be, they will be better able than at present to understand why. Defining criteria for personal maturity is a challenging task. Such issues as the capacity to reflect on oneself and learn from mistakes, to challenge authority in a constructive way, to be able to resolve conflict, to be reliable and consistent, and to have a balanced attitude towards work and leisure would be among the essential qualities of a psychotherapist. Work in this area is an urgent task for psychotherapy councils.

Another important job for the training committee of a psychotherapy council should be to define clearly the levels of training required for each type of practice. At present, given the lack of agreed standards, there are no clear guidelines as to who should be allowed to practise what sort of therapy. For example, many psychoanalysts strongly resist being classified with, say, psychoanalytic psychotherapists from some training organizations who, they correctly point out, generally have less intensive training than themselves; some analysts, in turn, could be accused of a false superiority based as much on guild protectionism and snobbery as on legitimate expertise.

The different types of psychotherapy training need to be placed on a more coherent and rational footing. In Britain, for example, such training is available in a number of different forms.

First, it may be part of a professional training—for instance, of psychiatrists and psychologists. For some, as we have pointed out, this may be little more than a smattering, while others go on to an extensive four-year programme, such as that received by senior psychiatric trainees in psychotherapy (who will then become consultant psychotherapists—see Glossary), or the unique programme at the Tavistock Clinic in London, which trains psychologists, social workers, and psychiatrists in analytic psychotherapy.

Second, there are the privately run training courses of the various psychoanalytic and psychotherapy organizations. These vary greatly in quality, length, and depth and are at present subject to no external scrutiny. Some are highly respectable and reputable, others much less so. The majority offer training in one particular branch of psychotherapy only (psychoanalysis, family therapy, group analysis).

Finally, there are some university-based diploma and masters courses; these, too, are variable but tend to offer a broad theoretical and practical experience in psychotherapy, spanning more than one branch. They may, however, lack the depth offered by some specialized training organizations.

There is no simple way of knowing what training an individual who claims to be a "trained psychotherapist" has received, other than anecdotal knowledge gleaned from particular courses.

In our view, a range of established, inspected, and accredited psychotherapy trainings should be available which equip candidates to work with a variety of different patients, in different settings, and with different techniques (see chapter four). A fully qualified professional psychotherapist should, alongside her own special interest, be conversant with the range of psychotherapies, in order to be able to assess a patient's needs and match them to an appropriate therapy.

Trainings vary according to their depth and breadth. Discussion of the former may be based on Cawley's distinction between different *levels* of psychotherapy (Cawley, 1977) which, together with a recent updating (NHSE, 1996), can be adapted to the question of training as follows:

(A) *Basic training* in counselling and simple behavioural techniques, which should be available to all members of any helping profession. Within the NHS, Level A psychotherapy is often part of a package of treatment that may include medication, attendance at a Day Hospital, and so forth.

(B) *Professional training* in psychotherapy as *part* of training in medicine, psychology, or social work. Professionals such as psychologists often offer an eclectic client-oriented therapy as part of their generic work within the NHS or privately.

(C) *Specialist training* in one particular branch of psychotherapy, such as psychoanalysis, cognitive therapy, family therapy, or psychodrama. Here the patient is offered formal psychotherapy in a specific modality.

We would also emphasize the need for trainings that provide breadth as well as depth to psychotherapeutic skills. These might be termed *general trainings* and would be broad-based in three ways:

(i) theoretically—with a grounding in the theoretical foundations of psychotherapy—philosophical, scientific, and aesthetic;

(ii) in its approach to practice: offering training in the range and evaluation of the different psychotherapies;

(iii) in its ability to offer psychotherapeutic experiences in different settings, for example in hospitals, general practices, social service departments, and schools.

The development of psychotherapy courses offering such general training is, in our view, an essential part of the kind of professionalization of psychotherapy that we are advocating; at present, such courses are conspicuously rare.

From a sociological point of view, there is a need for more general training, because the knowledge base upon which a profession, as opposed to an occupation, rests, is always broader and deeper than would be needed simply to carry out the technical aspects of professional activities. As Goode (1960) points out, if restaurant-waiting were to become a profession, its inceptors would be required to have degrees in food science!

From the point of view of the development of the profession, there are two main reasons for the encouragement of general courses, based preferably in universities. First, without them, the cross-fertilization between different branches of psychotherapy that is essential for the development of the subject is less likely to occur. Second, psychotherapists with a general training are needed for the wider dissemination and democratization of psychotherapy (see chapters four and five). To achieve these aims, there is a need for the state greatly to continue to expand its funding for psychotherapy training courses in colleges and universities. These would then, as a few are at present, be in a position to confer formal qualifications such as certificates, diplomas, and postgraduate degrees in psychotherapy on successful candidates.

A further proposal that could lead to more broadly educated psychotherapists, and away from rigid all-or-nothing types of training, would be a system of "credits" that a trainee would need to gain in order to become fully registered. These could be acquired from different courses and, if necessary, at different times. Thus, analytic psychotherapists might be required to gain one "minor" credit in cognitive therapy, and vice versa, and trainees could perhaps gain their "supervision" credit—a mark of their ability to offer supervision in psychotherapy—two or three years after acquiring their "seminar" credit.

The deployment of psychotherapists

One of the main themes of this book has been the need to widen the availability of psychotherapy.

The inadequacies and inequity of the British National Health Service are often highlighted by waiting-list figures for routine operations like hernia repair and treatment of varicose veins. These cause discomfort and restrictions and, if complications arise, mean potentially dangerous emergency surgery. The harm suffered by potential patients denied psychotherapy is at least as great as that endured by hernia patients faced with interminable waits for surgery: there is a comparable risk of a potentially fatal crisis, and the costs of treatment may well be comparable too.

In calling for a greater deployment of psychotherapy services to deal with mental distress, we are making a no more extravagant demand than those who (rightly) see the untardy provision of surgery for those in need as one hallmark of a civilized society.

Our demands have less urgency in some countries than in others. In Germany, for example, there are already Departments of Psychosomatic Medicine and Psychotherapy associated with medical schools in most major towns. These offer psychotherapy services to patients with psychosomatic and neurotic disorders and are staffed and funded on a scale that is unthinkable in the minuscule "psychotherapy departments" of British medical schools and hospitals, many of which are staffed on a part-time or voluntary basis.

Until psychotherapy is properly funded, there will be a serious problem about whether to concentrate scarce resources on a few highly trained therapists who will make their impact mainly as teachers and trainers of others, or to aim for a larger number of less highly trained psychotherapists who may have a greater immediate impact on the population.

Third World countries face comparable dilemmas in trying to develop their health services. Should they invest in expensive medical schools that will produce a small number of doctors who, through their teaching, will produce a "multiplier effect" and, through their special skill in treating serious disease, might improve the overall morale of the population but who may, once trained, emigrate or go into private practice? Or should they put the emphasis on "bare-foot doctors", who reach the remotest villages but cannot cope with serious cases?

The introduction of broad-based general psychotherapy trainings may go some way towards solving this dilemma by introducing a new type of psychotherapist who could work alongside both the specialist therapists like psychoanalysts, and the more versatile but less highly trained therapists, such as the nurse therapists. A broader approach to training would, we believe, generate an appreciation among psychotherapists of the need for much wider deployment, and of the necessity to put pressure on governments and other fund-giving agencies to provide finance.

How many psychotherapists? What would be the cost?

A detailed discussion of the funding of psychotherapy training and deployment is beyond the scope of this book and would, in any case, run the risk of being too parochial to be of any general significance. We have repeatedly made three general points: more psychotherapists are needed; this costs money; they need to be more equitably distributed. As an example, we may take the British Royal College of Psychiatrists' estimate that a minimum of one consultant psychotherapist is needed for every 200,000 members of the adult population (Royal College of Psychiatrists, 1975). In the United Kingdom, the figure is about 1:300,000 (Royal College of Psychiatrists, 1995), an average that masks the fact that in some regions the ratio is much lower. The Royal College also recommends (Royal College of Psychiatrists, 1988) a core team of at least three psychotherapists for each health district—that is, for about each 200,000 of the population. One of the team should be a medical psychotherapist (consultant psychotherapist), another should be a professional with specialist training (for instance, a psychologist), and the third might be a professional psychotherapist, not necessarily a doctor or a psychologist.

This would mean that, over the next twenty years or so, a large number of psychotherapists would need to be trained in the United Kingdom in addition to those who have already been trained. There will also be a need to provide continuing education and training for established core professionals. This translation of hopes and values into numbers immediately raises the question of costs and benefits.

We have already touched on this topic in chapter two. Here we consider two aspects only. The first concerns the individual patient. We have argued repeatedly that the scarcity of state-funded psychotherapy means that many patients who could benefit are excluded from treatment. We have also suggested that, even where public funds are available, potential patients are excluded by the selection process and the inflexible approach of practitioners. The rewards of being a psychotherapist extend beyond remuneration, and psychotherapists may tend to seek out "YAVIs" (young, attractive, verbal, intelligent, successful) patients to work with, thereby excluding some who are the most deserving of help. Some form of positive discrimination in favour of "difficult" and disadvantaged patients is needed.

General practitioners are given special allowances for working in deprived inner-city areas. There are already a few psychotherapy schemes in deprived areas, funded mainly by local authorities and voluntary agencies, and we believe that they should be encouraged. Where a state-run medical insurance scheme operates, as for example, in Canada and Germany (Thoma & Kachele, 1987), psychotherapists can be paid more for treating "difficult" patients with certain diagnostic and socioeconomic characteristics—for example, those who have had psychiatric diagnoses, and the unemployed. This arrangement is not dissimilar to the system of remuneration of dentists, who are reimbursed by the state for complicated work with poor patients. Private and voluntary sector psychotherapy schemes could be encouraged to extend already existing "Robin Hood"-type fees, in which the better-off subsidize the less well-off by paying more. A psychotherapy council would have the responsibility of fostering such arrangements.

The second issue, and a fundamental one for the fellow "impossible profession"—government—is the question of the costs of training and paying for the extra psychotherapists. There are too many uncertainties for an accurate cost–benefit analysis of public investment in psychotherapy to be established. As discussed in chapter two, a significant expansion of psychotherapy services would undoubtedly produce "hard" benefits, including a reduction in the bill for tranquillizers and anti-depressants, and lessen the burden on health and welfare services. "Soft" benefits, like improved quality of relationships and enhanced emotional autonomy and self-esteem, only rarely enter the equations of economists and politicians. The costs of training and funding the number of psychotherapists required would be considerable, but still a tiny amount when compared, say, with the cost of the Trident missile system or the NHS drugs bill. But whether expanding psychotherapy represents a "bargain" or a "waste of money" is not simply an empirical question and must ultimately be determined by the kind of moral and political evaluation in which we have been engaging throughout this book. It may be that a modern society that seeks to be liberal and democratic cannot afford *not* to invest substantially in psychotherapy.

CHAPTER ELEVEN

Epilogue:
the future of psychotherapy

Throughout this book we have returned repeatedly to the idea of autonomy. Autonomy, as we have characterized it, implies personal independence, emotional freedom, and the capacity to form satisfying relationships. Understood in this way, autonomy is one of the most valuable goals that psychotherapy can help its beneficiaries to achieve.

By focusing as we have on autonomy, we could perhaps be accused of neglecting other goals that embody the values of many psychotherapists. We have said little about the relation between psychotherapy's emphasis on childhood experience and the Christian tradition of reverence for innocence and simplicity. We have touched only lightly on the role of imagination and play in psychotherapy, nor have we related these to the heritage of Romanticism. We have only glancingly referred to the Kleinian emphasis on renunciation, suffering, and deferment of pleasures, nor have we related these to the tradition of radical dissent within Lutheran and puritan Christianity. We have barely mentioned concepts such as non-attachment (Holmes, 1996) and enlightenment, or their secular equivalents which include irony and humour, where the influence of Eastern philosophy and religion has made its impact on psychotherapy. We have said nothing of the connections between Judaism and psychoanalysis.

We have resisted the idea of psychotherapy as a secularized religion and have placed autonomy at the centre of the psychotherapeutic stage for three main reasons. First, because we see autonomy as a fundamental value from which many other values can be derived, including some that might be considered religious. Second, because autonomy as a value has long been recognized in Western political and philosophical thought. Third, because we see respect for autonomy as a unifying assumption shared by most psychotherapists of whatever persuasion.

There could, however, be dangers in relying simply on an unanalysed appeal to autonomy. Autonomy, like peace and freedom, is something whose value everyone will readily acknowledge. The flexibility of the concept potentially allows it to be seized on by proponents of radically different political persuasions to justify quite contrary policies and objectives, all in the name of "autonomy". Appeals to "autonomy" have, for example, been used by conservative libertarians to endorse the abolition of state "interference" with the free market, and by socialist political economists to justify restrictions on the power of monopolies to "force" consumers to trade on unacceptable terms. At an individual level, extreme selfishness and devil-take-the-hindmost attitudes are justified in the name of "autonomy", just as much as the emotional emancipation based on self-knowledge, relatedness, and concern, which psychotherapists advocate.

"Autonomy", it seems, is an "essentially contested concept": while autonomy is, everyone agrees, desirable, defenders of different political persuasions will seek to define it in such a way as to be able to show that their political programme is the only, or at least the best, way of promoting autonomy, and nobody can prove that their opponent's conception is mistaken. We concede that there is no one *true* meaning or Platonic Form of "autonomy", but it does not follow from this that use of the concept is vacuous. We have not appealed to "autonomy" *simpliciter*, but have described a particular conception of autonomy by reference to which the values of psychotherapy may be judged. The conception that we have been working with is, we believe, one that fits well with the liberal democratic tradition of John Stuart Mill, emphasizing the importance of an active engagement with the world based on a love of truth. It also incorporates psycho-therapeutic insights into the nature, complexity, and causes of emotional disturbance. It is, essentially, a liberal democratic conception which has been enriched by psychological knowledge unavailable to the classical theorists of liberal democracy, all of whom pre-dated Freud. Our hope is that those who already accept a liberal democratic conception of autonomy will see that the psychotherapeutic conception we have presented fits well with it—is, indeed, a natural extension of it.

"Autonomy" in the psychotherapeutic sense does not mean extreme selfishness, nor a supposed independence from other people. The British psychoanalyst John Bowlby (1979) is especially critical of the tendency, even within psychotherapy, to overvalue independence and to see dependency as an undesirable relic of childishness that the mature individual can, with therapeutic help, outgrow (Holmes, 1993). He sees mutuality and interdependence as biological and social necessities, and the process of psychotherapy not as an escape from all dependency, but as a replacement of compulsive dependency ("anxious attachment") with secure attachments that then form the basis of autonomous curiosity and creativity.

As pointed out in chapter three, the original (political) meaning of *autonomia* was not complete independence, but self-government, control over one's own affairs. The concept of "autonomy" has, certainly since the eighteenth century, been extended to the individual sphere. The distinctive contribution of psychotherapy to the development of the concept has been to show how individuals may lack control of their own lives, not just vis-à-vis society but in relation to their own internal states, and how self-knowledge and the internalization of good relationships ("good internal objects") may provide an important route to overcoming heteronomy.

Psychotherapeutic autonomy is thus more "positive" than Isaiah Berlin's "negative" conception of liberty (lack of state interference), but more "negative" than his full-blown "positive" conception (where liberty is equated with instantiations of a particular ideal of human perfection: Berlin, 1969). Psychotherapeutic autonomy is pluralistic in that it aims to help people to find and follow their *own* various goals and desires, without imposing any particular view of what is right upon them. Part of the process of therapy is helping people to recognize whether a particular decision or course of action feels right for *them*. The firm but non-coercive setting of therapy, the central importance of the relationship with the therapist, and the gradual internalization of both are the basis upon which patients may become able to make more autonomous choices.

Good psychotherapy emphasizes both the need for "holding" and maturation, and the value of exploration and self-discovery. Ethical problems arise when one or the other is missing. When psychotherapy repudiates the importance of providing a secure setting for maturation, and denies patients' needs for dependency, it runs the risk of degenerating into an irresponsible pastime. When it forgets the importance of letting patients discover and choose for themselves, it is in danger of *creating* unhealthy dependency rather than helping people to overcome it, and at worst of becoming a moralizing instrument of social control.

We have argued persistently for a broader and more just distribution of psychotherapy, which is at present largely available only to the well-off. As we see it, social injustice undermines autonomy in a society. We cannot accept Philip Rieff's view that "psychoanalytically speaking, there were free slaves in Athens, as there are enslaved citizens in New York" (Rieff, 1979). Emotional autonomy in conditions of political enslavement or social deprivation will not be fully realized, since material lack severely restricts the individual's opportunities for psychological development. In conditions of deprivation, emotional autonomy—which, we have argued, psychotherapy is capable of enhancing—is only a first step towards a wider emancipation and should not be seen as itself the ultimate goal. We are opposed to "Nirvanist", hedonistic psychotherapies for the rich, just as much as to the abuse of behavioural psychotherapy as a covert form of political control for the poor.

We have argued that, for psychotherapy to be equitable and ethical, it needs to organize itself into a profession. This means that psychotherapy will have to surrender a portion of its freedom: the particular form of autonomy that comes from being an outsider, unrecognized, and free from interference. But this, as we see it, is a price worth paying for becoming able to play a far more significant and beneficial social role. As we have pointed out, this move would not be without its own dangers. Many psychotherapists prefer to pursue spiritual rather than temporal power and fear that psychotherapy may lose its inherent subversiveness if incorporated, however peripherally, within the state apparatus. Professions, sadly, have a well-deserved reputation for being self-serving rather than meeting public need (Joseph, 1985).

Nevertheless, we *do* believe that psychotherapy should become a profession—for if psychotherapy is to flourish, it needs to be valued and supported by society, and becoming a profession is a necessary step towards this objective.

Donald Winnicott's phrase "there is no such thing as a baby"— that is, there is only a baby–mother couple—captures the importance of relationships and initial dependency for human survival (Winnicott, 1965). A baby that is not nurtured by a mother or mother-substitute will soon die. The same could be said of the residual emotional "baby" that persists through life and, as Heinz Kohut (1984) also argues, needs to be held and recognized in intimate relationships at whatever age. It is one of the functions of the psychotherapeutic relationship to provide such recognition and holding, without which there is a danger of emotional and spiritual death—and certainly no prospect of emotional autonomy.

In an analogous way it could be argued that just as babies cannot survive without mothers, so, too, institutions such as psychotherapy are ultimately unlikely to prosper without recognition by, and support from, *society*. Winnicott's insight, when applied to institutions, is in sharp contrast to the radical individualist view: "There is no such thing as society—only individuals and families." Although in a sense it is true that society is composed of a set of individuals, this individualist statement is misleading in that it obscures the interdependence of individuals and the fact that attempts to explain social change simply in terms of the intentional actions of individuals are inadequate.

If psychotherapy is to make the substantial contribution to human well-being that we think it should, it will need *societal* support and recognition, which go beyond individual action. Until psychotherapy becomes a profession, such support and recognition are unlikely to be forthcoming.

Another important connotation of the word "society" is the sense of "community". The claim that society does not exist is sometimes part of a strategy for avoiding a sense of responsibility for those in need, and for accepting the view that all state interventions are *ipso facto* a violation of personal autonomy.

The psychotherapeutic conception of autonomy which we advocate recognizes *both* the emotional interdependence of individuals within families *and* the importance of a wider sense of community at a societal level. The view that society does not exist leads to denial at a social level: denial of collective guilt, of the casualties produced by social structures, of social aggression. Psychotherapy's pursuit of autonomy, on the other hand, is based on the undoing of denial, on recognizing the importance of facing aggression, pain, loss, and handicap at a personal level and, by extension, within society.

The values of psychotherapy are, then, radically different from those that actually prevail in many contemporary Western societies. Given this, how can we be so sanguine in our advocacy of a psychotherapy profession? Is there the remotest chance that the changes that we advocate will come about?

We are convinced, and hope we have convinced our readers, of the usefulness and importance of psychotherapy. But it would be extremely naive if we were to think that social change, even the modest one that we are advocating, will come about through reasoned argument alone. Within the present climate of opinion, governments are especially unlikely to be willing to finance a new large expenditure on a caring profession such as psychotherapy.

In the last decade, there has been a marked shift in governmental policies throughout the liberal democracies away from Keynesian economics and welfarism. Within such a climate, it is especially difficult to secure public investment in projects that have little immediate tangible pay-off. As many of the benefits of psychotherapy are long-term and intangible, and many of the values of psychotherapy conflict with those of the prevailing *mores*, how *could* the political climate be right for expanding psychotherapy so as to benefit those who need it but for whom it is currently unavailable?

The case for expansion is, however, far from hopeless. History contains many examples of morally desirable social changes introduced primarily for reasons other than the manifest moral justifications that were brought forward in their support.

As we mentioned in our comparison between psychotherapy now and education in the middle of the nineteenth century, the introduction of universal education in Britain came about not, as one might think, primarily out of a concern for the educational welfare of children, but for a combination of other reasons—to do with fears about lawlessness on the streets and the threat posed by low-waged children to the employment prospects of adult women and men.

A similar process may lead to the advancement of psychotherapy for the following reasons.

In Western countries over the next few decades, there is likely to be a shift away from "Fordist" mass-production based on assembly lines and manned by unskilled or semi-skilled labour, towards highly skilled, individualist, "post-Fordist" work practices. These require a high degree of individual decision-making, independence, and emotional maturity on the part of the worker. The capacity of psychotherapy to enhance individuation and autonomy may come to be valued not as an end in itself, but as a necessary part of the productive process in an affluent society.

Alongside, and perhaps partly as a result of, this increasing affluence, there is growing evidence of widespread disaffection and unhappiness within industrialized societies. The evidence for this includes, for example, long-term high levels of unemployment, especially among the young, and escalating divorce and crime figures. Half of all marriages in the United States and one third in the United Kingdom now end in divorce; in Britain, the crime rate has increased by over 50 per cent during the last decade; in the United States, 25 per cent of all children and 60 per cent of black children are brought up in one-parent families. Child abuse has risen dramatically. Personal unhappiness, social disaffection, and intolerance have not been reduced as material wealth has increased.

Such social disintegration is harmful to society as a whole, not just to those who are themselves disaffected or dissatisfied. To the extent that this is true, there are reasons of enlightened self-interest—even for those doing well out of such societies—for seeking to prevent, or at least reduce, it.

As discussed in chapter five, one possible response to such problems is to find ways of helping people to survive, through various forms of denial, without facing up to the situation that causes the pain or disaffection. This is given social expression in the wide use of tranquillizing drugs, but already this "solution" is beginning to be found wanting. There is widespread recognition that drugs like Valium, because of intoxication and addiction, can cause more problems than they solve. Prozac, an antidepressant, can, when appropriately prescribed, be a useful drug, but it is often given out indiscriminately in a response to distress that would be far better dealt with by counselling or psychotherapy. Psychotherapy offers a direct alternative to tranquillizers, as well as providing an opportunity to look at the causes of unhappiness and anxiety and therefore, at least in theory, offering some possibility of prevention. It is quite possible, then, that the pressures of modern society and the shortcomings of drug therapy will mean that psychotherapy is the most efficient (even within the narrow terms of monetarist economics) way of addressing the dissatisfaction and unhappiness caused by social disintegration. This would provide psychotherapy, especially if it accepts the need for brief evaluated treatments, with an opportunity for advancement.

Such a development would not be without its dangers. Brief symptom-orientated psychotherapy can, at its worst, offer little more than short-term solutions to problems that require more sustained and less unrealistically optimistic solutions. As Good warns:

> Brief psychotherapy is symbolic of the modern age in which we do everything intensely and quickly. Is it really surprising that therapy can be so short when we eat on the run, have sex in the car, expect fortunes overnight, and fight world wars in minutes? [Good, 1987]

Good's warning points to further levels of social threat far more menacing to Western society than even the breakdown of traditional patterns of work and family life, and here psychotherapy may also have a significant part to play. At the extreme are the threats of global calamity, which include the ever-widening gap between rich and poor nations, the increasing destruction of the environment, and the ever-present possibility of nuclear war. At an intermediate level are social traumas characterized by massive loss. Over the past few years these have included, among countless others, the earthquake in Armenia; environmental disasters such as Chernobyl and Bhopal; the Zeebrugge and Philippines ferry disasters; the famines in Northeast and Central Africa; the Bangladesh floods; Rwandan genocide; and the devastation caused by the AIDS epidemic, especially in developing countries. However remote—or close to home—these traumas are, their imagery is, especially through television, flashed around the world into the conscious and unconscious minds of the population, to be followed seconds later by advertisements appealing to wholly incompatible emotions—encouraging the consumption of fast cars, expensive homes, and exotic holidays by happily married couples with model children and friends.

It is here that psychotherapy has an important contribution to make, for, uniquely, psychotherapy—and analytic approaches in particular—have the capacity to articulate the impact of social events at a personal level. The concepts of repression and denial of grief, loss, and mourning, of recovery and reparation, have roots in psychoanalysis. Attachment theory provides a basis for a politics based more in community than individualism, one that emphasizes the absolute centrality of social bonds rather than the illusory freedoms of naked capitalism (Kraemer & Roberts, 1996).

Medicine has always provided an indispensable metaphor for the affliction, diagnosis, and treatment of social ills: a recent British Prime Minister, for example, celebrated becoming the longest-serving premier of the century by saying that during her administration the *remedy* had been found for the "British *disease*". The concepts of psychotherapy may well be needed to characterize the experience of life in the next hundred years. On the positive side, what is distinctive of our society is independence and autonomy. On the negative side are not just the loss of life, but the loss of a meaning for life; what is suffered is not so much physical pain, but the mental pain of anxiety and depression; and what is feared as much as illness and death is dying alone surrounded by strangers. To these experiences, psychotherapy can give both a voice and succour.

One of the main themes of this book has been an exploration of the links between autonomy—so central to the tradition of philosophical and political thought in Western democracies—and the practice of psychotherapy. The conception of autonomy with which we have been working embraces self-knowledge, facing up to reality, acknowledgement of the need for deep personal relationships. The autonomy of individuals need not be in irreconcilable conflict with the society or community that nurtures them—in a better society it would not be.

One aspect of this vision is the belief that psychotherapy will advance on its own terms, both as an effective treatment for neurosis and, at a more profound level, as one means by which people may be helped to face, to overcome where necessary, or to realize their deepest longings. We also believe, ironically, that the strains of any society based on the alternative view of autonomy, in which individualism, competitiveness, and isolationism are valued as ends in themselves, will ultimately generate a need for assistance from psychotherapy. First, because society needs autonomous workers, not drones. Second, because of a phenomenon with which psychotherapists are all too familiar: the "return of the repressed", that tragic aspect of human nature by which, despite the best hopes and intentions, aspects of the self that have been neglected, denied, or swept aside return with renewed vigour to claim attention. As personal dissatisfaction and disaster haunt an increasingly atomized society, psychotherapy may be invited, even from the most unlikely quarters, to help.

For these reasons, we see an increasing recognition of the values of psychotherapy not just as desirable, but as inevitable.

GLOSSARY

Terms and titles within psychotherapy can be confusing. The following list is not intended to be exhaustive, but merely to help orientate the uninitiated. The interested reader should consult Bloch, Kovel, or Rycroft for further clarification:

S. Bloch, *What Is Psychotherapy?* (Oxford: Oxford University Press, 1979).

J. Kovel, *A Complete Guide to Therapy: From Psychoanalysis to Behaviour Modification* (Harmondsworth: Penguin, 1978).

C. Rycroft, *A Critical Dictionary of Psychoanalysis* (Harmondsworth: Penguin, new edition 1997).

In such a shifting and contentious field as psychotherapy, definitions and distinctions are liable to inaccuracy and, where incorrect or exclusive, to cause offence. We are aware of these dangers and do not pretend to offer *the* correct set of definitions and distinctions. The prime purpose of this glossary is to explain to the reader how *we* have categorized and defined the various terms in this book.

Professionals

child psychotherapist Psychoanalytic psychotherapist who works with children. Unconscious attitudes, desires, and emotions are explored with the child through play and drawings, rather than primarily through words. Child psychotherapy was pioneered by Freud's daughter Anna, and by Melanie Klein.

clinical psychologist Psychology graduate who has undergone a three-year postgraduate training in methods of psychological treatment, especially as applied to medicine, psychiatry, and mental handicap. Clinical psychologists lay great emphasis on scientific evaluation of treatment and tend, in general, to be cognitive-behavioural and eclectic rather than analytic in orientation.

consultant psychotherapist In the United Kingdom, a medical graduate who has undergone three years of training in psychiatry and a further three years of specialist psychotherapy training. Many are also psychoanalysts or have had psychoanalytic training. Consultant psychotherapists tend to be analytic rather than behavioural in orientation.

counsellor Counselling is usually seen as a basic form of psychotherapy (or psychotherapy as a sophisticated form of counselling!). The theoretical basis of counselling is the work of Carl Rogers, who advocated a theory-free encounter with the reality of the client (see below, Rogerian therapy). Counsellors are accredited by The British Association of Counsellors (BAC)

Jungian analyst (analytical psychologist) Follower of the school of Carl Jung, who has undergone a three- to four-year training, comprising personal therapy, supervised practice, and theoretical seminars. If trained in Zurich ("Zurich" analyst), tends to be interested in archetypes and the collective unconscious. More pragmatic British-trained Jungian analysts are members of the Society for Analytical Psychology (SAP).

"lay" analyst Now almost obsolete term used in the early days of psychoanalysis to refer to non-medical psychoanalysts. The majority of non-medical psychoanalysts now have a professional qualification (e.g. in psychology or social work) and are therefore not members of the laity.

psychiatrist Medical graduate who has undertaken at least three years of general training in the diagnosis and treatment of mental illness. Consultant psychiatrists in the United Kingdom will have undertaken a further four years of specialist training. The majority of psychiatrists receive some psychotherapy training, both analytic and behavioural, but in the United Kingdom, as opposed to Australasia and some states in the United States of America, this is considered desirable but not mandatory.

psychoanalyst Member or associate member of a psychoanalytical society affiliated to the International Psychoanalytical Association, which was set up by Freud and his followers in the 1920s. Training takes three to four years and comprises personal analysis five times a week, two cases treated five times a week under supervision, and theoretical seminars. Psychoanalysts in Britain are divided into one of three streams: followers of Melanie Klein, adherents to Freud's own views ("Contemporary Freudian"), and those who are not exclusively committed to either ("Independent" or "middle" group). May be member of BCP or UKCP.

psychologist Strictly speaking, a psychology graduate. Almost all clinical psychologists, and some psychiatrists, are psychology graduates. Often used by the general public, incorrectly, as a synonym for clinical psychologist.

psychotherapist Generic term for those who use psychological methods to alleviate mental distress or illness. Psychotherapists include psychologists, psychiatrists, and psychoanalysts and, at present, practitioners with no formal qualifications who assume the title (see chapter ten). Most reputable psychotherapists are registered, via their training organization, through the UKCP.

Therapies ("schools")

behaviour therapy Therapy based on the theories of, among others, Pavlov, Wolpe, Watson, and Skinner, who see neurosis as a product of faulty conditioning. Behaviour therapy starts from the position that what needs to be changed for people in distress is *maladaptive behaviour* rather than thoughts or feelings. A patient with agoraphobia, for example, will be encouraged by the therapist to go out of the house with a companion until she feels safe enough to venture out alone. Success is rewarded by praise, or perhaps by the patient buying herself a "treat" when she has overcome her fears, based on the principle of "operant conditioning" in which a previously feared stimulus becomes, through treatment, associated with reward rather than painful anxiety. Behaviour therapy is particularly effective for patients with fears and phobias (e.g. spider phobia) and for obsessional conditions such as compulsive cleaning or hand-washing.

cognitive behaviour therapy   Related to behaviour therapy, based on the ideas of George Kelly and Aaron Beck. Sees neurosis as a product of faulty "cognitions" (i.e. thoughts) and assumptions which need to be modified (by "cognitive restructuring") in therapy. A depressed person may, for instance, feel that her phone never rings because everyone hates her. The patient is invited by the therapist to challenge this view by alternative hypotheses—for example, that the phone is out of order, or that because she is depressed she has not contacted her friends and so they assume that she does not want to see them, or else has gone away.

dynamic psychotherapy   Variant of psychoanalytic or "Freudian" therapy. Based on the view that neurosis is the product of a "dynamic" of conflicting forces that permeate the patient's relationships, and that reach back to childhood. Conflicts arise between the demands of the "pleasure principle" (e.g. the need for intimacy) and those of the "reality principle" (in which children are, for example, exposed to traumas and adult whims over which they have no control). Neurosis may result from the immature ego's attempts to defend itself from the anxiety that this conflict produces. In therapy, the patient is made aware of these anxieties and traumas and of her *defences* against them.

Gestalt therapy   One of the new or "humanistic" therapies. Based on the idea that in neurosis the patient is repressing one part of the *whole* (translation of the German *"Gestalt"*) perceptual field, and that by reliving a painful experience wholeness can be restored. A bereaved person suffering from *persistent* "pathological grief" might be asked to "visualize" the dead person in an empty chair and speak to her as though she were actually present. The resulting catharsis of blocked feelings may allow the normal grieving process then to proceed. Gestalt therapy emphasizes the importance of *experiencing* feelings in sessions rather than *talking about* them.

hypnotherapy   Pre-dates Freud. Literally "sleep therapy". The patient is put into a state of deep relaxation in which she is especially receptive to the suggestions and influences of the therapist such that she abandon maladaptive behaviour patterns. In a hypnotic "trance", the patient may also relive, and perhaps overcome, childhood traumas. Contains elements of both behavioural and psychodynamic theories.

psychoanalysis   Classical Freudian therapy. The analyst is "opaque" and offers *interpretations*. The patient lies on a couch, tries to say whatever comes into her mind, recounts dreams, and normally attends for therapy five times a week over several years. Therapy proceeds through *insight*, and this comes mainly from *transference*, that is, reliving childhood relationships and traumas in the relationship with the analyst (see chapter six). In therapy, transferential feelings are interpreted, worked through, and resolved.

psychoanalytic psychotherapy   Variant of psychoanalysis, but less intense. For example, the patient usually attends only once or twice a week, and she sits in a chair rather than lying on a couch. Therapy may be "brief", no more than twenty sessions in all, or prolonged. The analysis of transference, and of dynamic factors—that is, defences and impulses—is used in the search for insight, meaning, mastery, and relief.

psychodrama   Initiated by Jacob Moreno. As in Gestalt therapy, the patient re-enacts painful experiences, in a group, with others in the group playing important *dramatis personae* from her past (including herself). Scenes can be re-examined, blocked emotions released, and alternative versions of the past reconsidered. Psychodrama works through catharsis and cognitive restructuring.

Rogerian therapy   Based on the "client-centred" approach of Carl Rogers. The main effort of the therapist is to empathize and identify with the patient. "Interpretations" are eschewed, since in Rogers' view they have a distancing effect. The therapist mainly tries to "reflect" back what the patient is saying, thinking, and feeling, so that it can be seen in a more objective light. According to Rogers, the three essential characteristics of a successful therapist are empathy, genuineness, and non-possessive warmth.

supportive psychotherapy   Closely related to Rogerian therapy, a low-key approach in which the patient's "defences" are, on the whole, shored up rather than challenged, and strengths rather than weaknesses emphasized. Suitable for very disturbed or disadvantaged patients whose self-esteem is so fragile that breakdown might result if offered a more active or powerful form of therapy.

systemic therapy   Basis of much family therapy, deriving from, among others, Gregory Bateson. Sees the family not as a collection of individuals but as a whole "system" with its own rules and structures which, when difficulties arise, becomes dysfunctional. In "healthy" families, for instance, there is a perceptible though permeable "sub-system boundary" between parents and children. A child with psychogenic asthma may spend every night in her parents' bed, thereby transgressing the parent–child boundary and so leading to a deterioration of the parents' sexual relationship. Parents who are not getting on may also unconsciously arouse anxiety in a child, thus leading to asthma, and so "invite" the child into their bed, thus leading to further deterioration in their relationship. Vicious circles such as these, in which the symptom (in this case, asthma) is both a cause and a consequence of family dysfunction, are what systemic therapists call "circular causality". Systemic therapists may try to break the vicious circles behaviourally—for example, by encouraging the parents firmly to take the child back to her own bed—or occasionally by *paradox* (see chapter eight), in which the parents might be shocked into a healthier relationship by the therapist suggesting that the child spends every night in their bed and that they abandon sexual contact altogether.

Arrangements

family therapy   More than one member of a family meeting with a therapist or therapists. Although most family therapists practise systemic therapy, family therapists may also adopt a psychoanalytic approach in which the therapist attends primarily to the underlying emotional life of the family members, rather than trying directly to change their behaviour or alter the family structure.

group therapy   At least two patients, who are not members of the same family, meeting with a therapist or therapists. A "small group" normally consists of four to ten members. A "large group", seen in some hospital psychiatric wards, has up to thirty members. "Group analysis" applies psychoanalytic principles to group therapy. A group that is very reliant on its therapist, for instance, would be seen as having a "group transference" of dependency, and interpretation of this might open up discussion of individual members' dependency needs and their fear of autonomy. Behaviourally oriented groups—for example, where a group of agoraphobic patients set tasks and work on problems together—are also widely used.

individual therapy   Literally, any therapeutic meeting in which one therapist meets one patient. Sometimes used as a shorthand for psychoanalytic psychotherapy.

marital therapy   A married couple meeting with a therapist or therapists. Behavioural marital therapy focuses on behaviours, cognitive marital therapy on shared assumptions, and analytic marital therapy on unconscious shared fears and projections of married couples.

REFERENCES

American Psychiatric Association (1985). *The Principles of Medical Ethics with Annotations Especially Applicable to Psychiatry.* Washington.

Appelbaum, P. S,. Lidz, C. W., & Meisel, A. (Eds.) (1987). *Informed Consent: Legal Theory and Clinical Practice.* New York: Oxford University Press.

Baker, J. (1987). *Arguing for Equality.* London: Verso.

Balint, M. (1957). *The Doctor, his Patient and the Illness.* London: Pitman.

Barker, C. (1983). The psychotherapist. In: N. T. Singleton (Ed.), *The Analysis of Real Skills: Social Skills.* Oxford: Oxford University Press.

Bateman, A., & Holmes, J. (1995). *Introduction to Psychoanalysis: Contemporary Theory and Practice.* London: Routledge.

Bentham, J. (1789). *The Principles of Morals and Legislation.* In: M. Warnock (Ed.), *Utilitarianism.* London: Fontana/Collins, 1962.

Berlin, I. (1969). Two concepts of liberty. In: *Four Essays on Liberty.* Oxford: Oxford University Press.

Bernstein, B. (1964). Social class, speech systems and psychotherapy. *British Journal of Sociology, 15*: 54–64.

Bettelheim, B. (1960). *The Informed Heart.* New York: Free Press.

Bettelheim, B. (1983). *Freud and Man's Soul.* London: Chatto & Windus.

Blass, R., & Simon, B. (1994). The value of the historical perspective to contemporary psychoanalysis: Freud's "seduction hypothesis". *International Journal of Psycho-Analysis, 75*: 677–694.

Bloch, S. (1981). The political misuse of psychiatry in the Soviet Union. In: S. Chodoff & P. Chodoff (Eds.), *Psychiatric Ethics*. Oxford: Oxford University Press.

Bloch, S. (1996). Ethics and Psychotherapy. *American Journal of Psychotherapy, 30*: 257–258.

Bok, S. (1978). *Secrets: On the Ethics of Concealment and Revelation*. Oxford: Oxford University Press.

Bornstein, R. (1993). Implicit perception, implicit memory, and the recovery of unconscious material in psychotherapy. *Journal of Nervous and Mental Disease, 181*: 337–344.

Bowlby, J. (1979). *The Making and Breaking of Affectional Bonds*. London: Tavistock.

Bowlby, J. (1988). Developmental psychiatry comes of age. *American Journal of Psychiatry, 145*: 1-10.

British Association for Social Work (1975). *A Code of Ethics for Social Work* (adopted at Annual General Meeting, Edinburgh). Reprinted in: D. Watson (Ed.), *A Code of Ethics for Social Work: The Second Step*. London: Routledge & Kegan Paul, 1985.

British Medical Association (1981). *The Handbook of Medical Ethics*. London.

British Psychological Society (1995). *Recovered Memories: Report of the Working Party of the BBS*. Leicester.

Brooks, N. (1988). Indications for coronary artery surgery. *Journal of the Royal College of Physicians of London, 22* (1): 23–27.

Brown, G., & Harris, T. (1978). *The Social Origins of Depression*. London: Tavistock.

Byng-Hall, J. (1995). *Rewriting Family Scripts*. London: Guilford Press.

Cade, B. (1979). The use of paradox in therapy. In: S. Walrond-Skinner (Ed.), *Family and Marital Psychotherapy: A Critical Approach*. London: Routledge & Kegan Paul.

Casement, P. (1985). *On Learning from the Patient*. London: Tavistock.

Cawley, R. (1977). The teaching of psychotherapy. *Association of University Teachers of Psychiatry Newsletter*, pp. 19–36.

Chadwick, P., & Birchwood, M. (1994). The omnipotence of voices: a cognitive approach to auditory hallucinations. *British Journal of Psychiatry, 164*: 190–201.

Chasseguet-Smirgel, J. (1985). *Creativity and Perversion*. London: Free Association Books.

Cheifetz, L. G. (1984). Framework violation in psychotherapy with clinic patients. In: J. Rawley (Ed.), *Listening and Interpreting: The Challenge of the Work of Robert Langs*. London: Jason Aronson.

Cioffi, F. (1970). Freud and the ideas of a pseudo-science. In: R. Borger & F. Cioffi (Eds.), *Explanation in the Behavioural Sciences*. Cambridge: Cambridge University Press.

City of Bradford Metropolitan District Council (1985). *Recruitment and Selection: Code of Practice*. Bradford.

Clarkson, P., & Pokorny, M. (1994). *The Handbook of Psychotherapy*. London: Routledge.

Coleman, V. (1985). *Life Without Tranquillisers: How to Survive Stress and Anxiety without Drugs*. London: Corgi.

Collier, A. (1987). The language of objectivity and the ethics of reframing. In: S. Walrond-Skinner & D. Watson (Eds.), *Ethical Issues in Family Therapy*. London: Routledge & Kegan Paul.

Cosin, B. R., Freeman, C. F., & Freeman, N. H. (1972). Critical empiricism criticised. *Journal of the Theory of Social Behaviour, 1* (2): 121–151. Reprinted in: R. Wollheim & J. Hopkins (Eds.), *Philosophical Essays on Freud*. Cambridge: Cambridge University Press, 1982.

Crowe, M. (1978). Conjoint marital therapy: a controlled outcome study. *Psychological Medicine, 8*: 623–636.

Daniels, N. (1985). *Just Health Care*. Cambridge: Cambridge University Press.

Davidson, D. (1980). Mental events and other essays. In: *Essays on Action and Events*. Oxford: Oxford University Press.

De Zuluetta, F. (1993). *From Pain to Violence*. London: Whurr.

Dolan, B., & Norton, K. (1996). *Perspective on the Henderson*. London: Henderson Publications.

Eagleton, T. (1985). *Critical Theory*. London: Verso.

Ellenberger, H. (1970). *The Discovery of the Unconscious*. New York: Basic Books.

Epstein, W. (1995). *The Illusion of Psychotherapy*. New Brunswick, NJ: Transaction Publishers.

Ernst, S., & Goodison, L. (1981). *In Our Own Hands: A Book of Self-Help Therapy*. London: Women's Press.

Eysenck, H. J. (1952). The effects of psychotherapy: an evaluation. *Journal of Consulting Psychology, 16*: 319–324.

Eysenck, H. J. (1983). An analysis of psychotherapy versus placebo studies. *Behaviour and Brain Sciences, 6*: 275–310.

Ferenczi, S. (1955). *Final Contributions to the Problems and Methods of Psycho-Analysis*. London: Hogarth. [Reprinted London: Karnac Books, 1994.]

Ferenczi, S. (1960). The further development of an active therapy in psychoanalysis. *Further Contributions to the Theory and Technique of Psychoanalysis*. London: Hogarth. [Reprinted London: Karnac Books, 1994.]

Foster, J. G. (1971). *Enquiry into the Practice and Effects of Scientology*. London: HMSO.

Frank, J. (1973). *Persuasion and Healing: A Comparative Study of Psychotherapy*. Baltimore: Johns Hopkins University Press.

Freud, S. (1887–1904). *The Complete Letters of Sigmund Freud to Wilhelm Fliess*. Cambridge, MA: Harvard University Press, 1985.

Freud, S. (1895d) (with Breuer, J.). *Studies on Hysteria, S.E., 20*.

Freud, S. (1896c). The aetiology of hysteria. *S.E., 3*.

Freud, S. (1899a). Screen memories. *S.E., 3*.

Freud, S. (1912b). The dynamics of transference. *S.E., 12*.

Freud, S. (1912e). Recommendations to physicians practising psychoanalysis. *S.E., 3*.

Freud, S. (1919a). Lines of advance in psychoanalytic therapy. *S.E., 17*.

Freud, S. (1923b). *The Ego and the Id. S.E., 19*.

Freud, S. (1925e). Resistances to psychoanalysis. *S.E., 19*.

Freud, S. (1926e). The question of lay analysis. *S.E., 20*.

Freud, S. (1930a). *Civilization and its Discontents*, trans. Joan Riviere, p. 117 footnote. Quoted in F. Cioffi, "Freud and the ideas of a pseudo-science", in: R. Borger & F. Cioffi (Eds.), *Explanation in the Behavioural Sciences*. Cambridge: Cambridge University Press, 1970.

Freud, S. (1937c). Analysis terminable and interminable. *S.E., 22*.

Freud, S. (1937d). Constructions in analysis. *S.E., 23*.

Freud, S. (1950). *Collected Papers*, trans. Joan Riviere, vol. 5, p. 231. Quoted in F. Cioffi, "Freud and the ideas of a pseudo-science", in: R. Borger & F. Cioffi (Eds.), *Explanation in the Behavioural Sciences*. Cambridge: Cambridge University Press, 1970.

Gabbard, G. (1996). Lessons to be learned from the study of sexual boundary violations. *American Journal of Psychotherapy, 50*: 311–322.

Garfield, S. L. (1986). Research in client variables in psychotherapy. In: S. L. Garfield & A. E. Bergin (Eds.), *Handbook of Psychotherapy and Behaviour Change*. Chichester: Wiley.

Garfield, S. L., & Bergin, A. E. (Eds.) (1986). *Handbook of Psychotherapy and Behaviour Change*. Chichester: Wiley.

Gartrell, N., et al. (1986). Psychiatrist-patient sexual contact. In: *American Journal of Psychiatry, 143* (9): 1126–1131.

Gartrell, N., et al. (1988). Psychiatric residents' sexual contact with educators and patients. *American Journal of Psychiatry, 145* (6): 690–694.

General Medical Council (1958). *Centenary of the General Medical Council: 1858–1958: A Brief History of the Council during Its First Hundred Years*. London.

George, S. (1979). *How the Other Half Dies*. Harmondsworth: Penguin.

Good, P. R. (1987). Brief therapy in the age of reagapeutics. *American Journal of Orthopsychiatry, 57* (1): 6–11.

Goode, W. (1960). Encroachment, charlatanism and the emerging profession: psychology, sociology and medicine. *American Sociological Review, 25*: 902–914.

Griffin, J. (1986). *Well-Being*. Oxford: Oxford University Press.

Grunbaum, A. (1984). *The Foundations of Psychoanalysis*. Berkeley, CA: University of California Press.

Halmos, P. (1965). *The Faith of the Counsellors*. London: Constable.

Hardin, G. (1979). Lifeboat earth: the case against helping the poor. In: J. Rachels (Ed.), *Moral Problems* (third series). New York: Harper & Row.

Heitler, J. B. (1976). Preparatory techniques in initiating expressive psychotherapy with lower-class unsophisticated patients. *Psychological Bulletin, 83*: 339–352.

Hinshelwood, R. (1995). The social relocation of personal identity as shown by psychoanalytic observations of splitting, projection and introjection. *Philosophy, Psychiatry, Psychology, 2*: 185–204.

HMSO (1980). *Behaviour modification*. Report of a joint working party to formulate ethical guidelines for the conduct of programmes of behaviour modification in the National Health Service: a consultative document with suggested guidelines. London.

Hogget, P., & Lonsada, J. (1985). Therapeutic intervention in working class communities. *Free Associations, 1*: 125–152.

Holland, S., & Holland, R. (1984). Depressed women: outposts of empire and castles of skin. In: B. Richards (Ed.), *Capitalism and Infancy*. London: Free Association Books.

Hollingshead, A. B., & Redlich, F. C. (1958). *Social Class and Mental Illness*. New York: Wiley.

Holmes, D. (1992). Race and transference in psychoanalysis and psychotherapy. *International Journal of Psycho-Analysis, 73*: 1–11.

Holmes, J. (1985). Family and individual therapy: comparisons and contrasts. *British Journal of Psychiatry, 147*: 668–676.

Holmes, J. (1986). Teaching the psychotherapeutic method: some literary parallels. *British Journal of Medical Psychology, 59*: 113–121.

Holmes, J. (1987). "Referral for psychotherapy: class, age and sex—bias in the selection process." Paper presented at the Society for Psychotherapy Research meeting, Ravenscar, Yorkshire.

Holmes, J. (1992). *Between Art and Science: Essays in Psychotherapy and Psychiatry*. London: Routledge.

Holmes, J. (1993). *John Bowlby and Attachment Theory*. London: Routlege.

Holmes, J. (1996). *Intimacy, Attachment, Autonomy: Using Attachment Theory in Adult Psychotherapy*. New York: Jason Aronson.

Holyroyd, J. C., & Brodsky, A. M. (1977). Attitudes and practices regarding erotic and nonerotic contacts with patients. *American Psychologist, 32*: 843–849.

Hume, D. (1739). *A Treatise of Human Nature*, Selby-Bigge edition. Oxford: Oxford University Press, 1960.

Hunt, M. (1985). Psychotherapy and psychiatric need. *British Journal of Psychiatry, 146*: 669–670.

Huxley, A. (1955). *Brave New World*. Harmondsworth: Penguin.

Illich, I. (1975). *Medical Nemesis: The Expropriation of Health*. London: Calder & Boyars.

Jacoby, R. (1975). *Social Amnesia: A Critique of Conformist Psychology from Adler to Laing*. Hassocks: Harvester Press.

Joseph, M. (1985). *Lawyers Can Seriously Damage Your Health*. London: Michael Joseph.

Kant, I. (1795). Groundwork of the metaphysics of morals. In: H. J. Paton, *The Moral Law*. London: Hutchinson, 1948.

Kant, I. (1798). On a supposed right to lie from altruistic motives. In: *Critique of Practical Reason and Other Writings in Moral Philosophy*, ed. and trans. Lewis White Beck. Chicago, IL: University of Chicago Press, 1949. Quoted in: S. Bok, *Lying: Moral Choice in Public and Private Life*. Hassocks: Harvester Press, 1978.

Karasu, T. B. (1981). Ethical aspects of psychotherapy. In: S. Bloch & P. Chodoff, *Psychiatric Ethics*. Oxford: Oxford University Press.

Karasu, T. B. (1986). The psychotherapies: benefits and limitations. *American Journal of Psychotherapy, 40* (3): 324–343.

Klerman, G. L. (1986). Drugs and psychotherapy. In: S. L. Garfield &

A. E. Bergin (Eds.), *Handbook of Psychotherapy and Behaviour Change*. Chichester: Wiley.

Kohon, G. (1984). Reflections on Dora: the case of hysteria. *International Journal of Psychoanalysis, 65*: 73–84.

Kohon, G. (1986). *The British School of Psychoanalysis: The Independent Tradition*. London: Free Association Books.

Kohut, H. (1984). *How Does Analysis Cure?* Chicago, IL: University of Chicago Press.

Kovel, J. (1978). *A Complete Guide to Therapy: From Psychoanalysis to Behaviour Modification*. Harmondsworth: Penguin.

Kraemer, S., & Roberts, J. (1996). *The Politics of Attachment*. London: Free Association Books.

Laing, R. D. (1960). *Self and Others*. London: Tavistock.

Lakin, M. (1988). *Ethical Issues in the Psychotherapies*. New York: Oxford University Press.

Lambert, M. J., Shapiro, D., & Bergin, A. E. (1986). The effectiveness of psychotherapy. In: S. L. Garfield & A. E. Bergin (Eds.), *Handbook of Psychotherapy and Behaviour Change*. Chichester: Wiley.

Lane, P., & Spruill, J. (1980). To tell or not to tell: the psychotherapist's dilemma. *Psychotherapy: Theory, Research and Practice, 17* (2): 202–209.

Leff, J., & Vaughn, C. (1984). *Expressed Emotion in Families: Its Significance for Mental Illness*. New York: Guilford Press.

Leff, J., Kuipers, L., & Berkowitz, R. (1982). A controlled trial of social intervention in the families of schizophrenic patients. *British Journal of Psychiatry, 141*: 121–134.

Lerner, B. (1972). *Therapy in the Ghetto*. Baltimore: Johns Hopkins University Press.

Lindley, R. (1986). *Autonomy*. London: Macmillan.

Lindley, R. (1987). Family therapy and respect for people. In: S. Walrond-Skinner & D. Watson (Eds.), *Ethical Issues in Family Therapy*. London: Routledge & Kegan Paul.

Lindley, R. (1988). Psychotherapy as essential care. In: G. Fairbairn & S. Fairbairn (Eds.), *Psychology, Ethics and Change*. London: Routledge & Kegan Paul.

Lindsay, D., & Read, J. (1994). Psychotherapy and memories of childhood sexual abuse: a cognitive perspective. *Applied Cognitive Psychology, 8*: 281–338.

Livingston Smith, D. (1991). *Hidden Conversations: The Communicative Critique and Reconstruction of Psychoanalysis*. London: Routledge.

Loftus, E. (1993). The reality of repressed memories. *American Psychologist, 48:* 518–537.

Lorion, R. P., & Felner, R. D. (1986). Research on mental health interventions with the disadvantaged. In: S. L. Garfield & A. E. Bergin (Eds.), *Handbook of Psychotherapy and Behaviour Change.* Chichester: Wiley.

Luborsky, L., et al. (1985). Therapist success and its determinants. *Archives of General Psychiatry, 42:* 602–611.

Luborsky, L., et al. (1986). Do therapists vary much in their success? Findings from four outcome studies. *American Journal of Orthopsychiatry, 56* (4): 501–513.

Luborsky, L., Singer, B., & Luborsky, B. (1975). Comparative studies of psychotherapies: is it true that "everyone has won and all must have prizes"? *Archives of General Psychiatry, 32:* 995–1008.

Mahler, M. (1969). *On Human Symbiosis and the Vicissitudes of Individualism.* London: Hogarth.

Malan, D. (1963). *A Study of Brief Psychotherapy.* London: Tavistock.

Marcuse, H. (1966). *Eros and Civilisation.* Boston: Beacon Press.

Mays, D. T., & Frank, C. M. (1985). *Negative Outcome in Psychotherapy and What to Do About It.* New York: Springer.

McGrath, G., & Lowson, K. (1986). Assessing the benefits of psychotherapy: the economic approach. *British Journal of Psychiatry, 150:* 65–71.

Mill, J. S.(1861). *Utilitarianism.* In: M. Warnock (Ed.), *Utilitarianism.* London: Fontana/Collins, 1962.

Miller, A. (1985). *Thou Shalt Not Be Aware.* London: Pluto.

Minuchin, S., et al. (1963). *Families of the Slums: An Exploration of Their Structure and Treatment.* New York: Basic Books.

Mollica, R. F., & Milic, M. (1986). Social class and psychiatric practice: a revision of the Hollingshead and Redlich model. *American Journal of Psychiatry, 143* (1): 12–17.

Mollon, P. (1996). *Multiple Selves, Multiple Voices. Working with Trauma, Violation and Dissociation.* Chichester: Wiley.

Mullen, P., Romans-Clarkson, S., Walton, V., & Herbison, P. (1993). Impact of sexual and physical abuse on women's mental health. *Lancet, 344:* 841–845.

Nagel, T. (1979). Death. In: T. Nagel, *Mortal Questions.* Cambridge: Cambridge University Press.

NHSE (1996). *Psychotherapy Services in England.* London: HMSO.

Nozick, R. (1974). *Anarchy, State and Utopia.* Oxford: Blackwell.

Parsons, T. (1951). *The Social System*. New York: Free Press.

Pedder, J. (1988). Lecture given to conference of the Association of University Teachers of Psychiatry, Oxford.

Pilkonis, P., et al. (1984). A comparative outcome study of individual, group and conjoint psychotherapy. *Archives of General Psychiatry, 41*: 431–437.

Poole, D., Lindsay, D., Memon, A., & Bull, R. (1995). Psychotherapy and the recovery of memories of childhood sexual abuse: US and British practitioners' opinions, practices and experiences. *Journal of Counselling and Clinical Psychology, 63*: 426–437.

Popper, K. (1960). *Logic of Scientific Discovery* (revised edn.). London: Hutchinson.

Reich, W. (1961). *The Function of the Orgasm*. New York: Farrar, Straus, & Giroux.

Reik, T. (1948). *Listening With The Third Ear*. New York: Farrar, Straus, & Giroux.

Rieff, P. (1979). *Freud: The Mind of the Moralist*, 3rd edn. London: University of Chicago Press.

Roazen, P. (1979). *Freud and His Followers*. London: Peregrine.

Rogers, C. R. (1957). The necessary and sufficient conditions of therapeutic personality change. *Journal of Consulting Psychology, 21*: 95–103.

Rosser, R. M., et al., (1987). Five-year follow up of patients treated with in-patient psychotherapy at the Cassel Hospital for Nervous Diseases. *Journal of the Royal Society of Medicine, 80*.

Roth, A. & Fonagy, P. (1996). *What Works for Whom*. New York: Guilford.

Royal College of Psychiatrists (1975). Norms for medical staffing of a psychotherapy service for a population of 200,000. *Bulletin of the Royal College of Psychiatrists* (October).

Royal College of Psychiatrists (1983). Report to council of the Royal College of Psychiatrists from the psychotherapy section executive committee. *Bulletin of the Royal College of Psychiatrists, 7* (10): 190–195.

Royal College of Psychiatrists (1988). *Future of Psychotherapy Services*. Report from psychotherapy section executive committee. Unpublished.

Royal College of Psychiatrists (1995). *Annual Census of Psychiatric Staffing, September 1994*. Unpublished.

Rustin, M., & Rustin, M. (1984). Relational preconditions of socialism. In: B. Richards (Ed.), *Capitalism and Infancy*. London: Free Association Books.

Rycroft, C. (1985). *Psychoanalysis and Beyond*. London: Chatto & Windus.

Ryle, A. (1982). *Psychotherapy: A Cognitive Integration of Theory and Practice*. London: Academic Press.

Sabbadini, A. (1992). "The truth is, sir, my nerves are bad." Reflections on Freud's case of Katerina. *British Journal of Psychotherapy*, 9: 157–168.

Samuels, S. (1993). *The Political Psyche*. London: Routledge.

Sandler, J. (1976). Counter-transference and role-responsiveness. *International Review of Psycho-analysis*, 3: 43–47.

Schafer, R. (1976). *A New Language for Psychoanalysis*. London: Yale University Press.

Schafer, R. (1983). *The Analytic Attitude*. New York: Basic Books.

Schank, R. (1982). *Dynamic Memory: A Theory of Reminding and Learning in Computers and People*. Cambridge: Cambridge University Press.

Schimek, J. (1985). Fact and fantasy in the seduction theory: a historical review. *Journal of the American Psychoanalytic Association*, 35: 937–965.

Schofield, W. (1965). *Psychotherapy: The Purchase of Friendship*. Cited in P. Halmos, *The Faith of the Counsellors*. London: Constable.

Segal, H. (1991). *Dream, Phantasy, Art*. London: Routledge.

Shapiro, D. (1995). Finding out about how psychotherapies help people change. *Psychotherapy Research*, 5: 1–21.

Shapiro, D., & Firth, J. (1987). Prescriptive v. exploratory therapy: outcomes of the Sheffield Psychotherapy Project. *British Journal of Psychiatry*, 15: 790–799.

Shepherd, M. (1979). Psychoanalysis, psychotherapy, and health services. *British Medical Journal*, 2: 1557–1559.

Sieghart, P. (1979). *Statutory Registration of Psychotherapists. A Report of a Profession's Joint Working Party*. Cambridge: E. E. Plumridge.

Singer, P. (1979). *Practical Ethics*. Cambridge: Cambridge University Press.

Sloane, R. B., et al. (1975). *Psychotherapy versus Behaviour Therapy*. Cambridge, MA: Harvard University Press.

Smith, M. L., Glass, G. V., & Miller, T. I. (1980). *The Benefits of Psychotherapy*. Baltimore, MD: Johns Hopkins University Press.

Spence, D. (1982). *Narrative Truth and Historical Truth: Meaning and Interpretation in Psychoanalysis*. New York: W. W. Norton.

Steiner, J. (1985). Psychotherapy under attack. *Lancet*, 1: 266–267.

Stiles, W. B., Shapiro, D. A., & Elliott, R. (1986). Are all psychotherapies equivalent? *American Psychologist*, 41 (2): 165–180.

Storr, A. (1979). *The Art of Psychotherapy*. London: Secker & Warburg.

Strachey, J. (1934). The nature of the therapeutic action of psychoanalysis. *International Journal of Psychoanalysis, 15*: 127–159.

Szasz, T. (1969). *The Ethics of Psychoanalysis: The Theory and Method of Autonomous Psychotherapy*. New York: Dell.

Szasz, T. (1973). *The Manufacture of Madness*. St Albans: Granada.

Szasz, T. (1974). *Law, Liberty and Psychiatry*. London: Routledge & Kegan Paul.

Szasz, T. (1979). *The Theology of Medicine*. Oxford: Oxford University Press.

Tarasoff decision: a decade later dilemma still faces psychotherapists (1987). *American Journal of Psychotherapy, 41* (2): 271–285.

Tarrier, N. (1988). Family involvement. *Current Opinion in Psychiatry, 1*: 201–205.

Taylor, F. K. (1987). Psychoanalysis: a philosophical critique. *Psychological Medicine, 17*: 557–560.

Thoma, H., & Kachele, H. (1987). *Psychoanalytic Practice*. London: Springer-Verlag.

Townsend, P., & Davidson, N. (1982). *Inequalities in Health: The Black Report*. Harmondsworth: Penguin.

Tuckett, D. (1995). The conceptualisation and communication of clinical facts in psychoanalysis. *International Journal of Psycho-Analysis, 76*: 653–661.

Tudor-Hart, J. (1971). The inverse care law. *Lancet, 1*: 405–412.

Tulving, E. (1985). How many memory systems are there? *American Psychologist, 40*: 385–398.

Walvin, J. (1982). *A Child's World: A Social History of English Childhood 1800–1914*. Harmondsworth: Penguin.

Watzlawick, P., Weakland, J., & Fisch, R. (1974). *Change: Principles of Problem Formation and Problem Resolution*. New York: W. W. Norton.

Webster, R. (1996). *Why Freud Was Wrong*. London: Fontana.

Weiskrantz, L. (1995). Comments on the Report of the Working Party of the British Psychological Society on "Recovered Memories". *The Therapist, 2*: 5–8.

Weissman, M., Sholomokas, D., & John, K. (1981). The assessment of social adjustment. *Archives of General Psychiatry, 38*: 1250–1258.

Wilkinson, G. (1986). Psychoanalysis and analytic psychotherapy in the National Health Service—a problem for medical ethics. *Journal of Medical Ethics, 12*: 87–90.

Williams, B. (1973). The idea of equality. Reprinted in: B. Williams, *Problems of the Self*. Cambridge: Cambridge University Press.

Wing, J. K., & Wing, L. (1970). Psychotherapy in the National Health Service: an operational study. *British Journal of Psychiatry, 116*: 556–563.

Winnicott, D. W. (1965). *The Maturational Process and the Facilitating Environment*. London: Hogarth. [Reprinted London: Karnac Books, 1994.]

INDEX

Printed in the United States
by Baker & Taylor Publisher Services

Printed in the United States
by Baker & Taylor Publisher Services